CONSENTING ADULTS ONLY

A novel of medicine, mayhem and a vicious
love triangle in modern-day Las Vegas

Lawrence Martin, M.D.

Copyright 2015 by Lawrence Martin, M.D.
Lakeside Press
Library of Congress number pending. LC case number is 1-2368717741
All material herein is copyright by the author with the exception of quoted song lyrics.

ISBN: 1879653052
ISBN 13: 9781879653054

Acknowledgments: Several people reviewed this manuscript in its various stages, and portions were critiqued in two writers groups in The Villages, Florida. A warm thank you to Katie Gerken, Marti Green, Danny Kaminsky, Dr. Ruth Martin, Bernard Martin, Sarah Miller, Deb Rhodes and Penny Strauss for their many insightful comments and suggestions.

Cover design by Judy Bullard
www.customebook**covers**.com

CONSENTING
ADULTS ONLY

Dedication: To my wife Ruth, a psychiatrist, who helped me get the psychology right. If anything in that area is wrong, it's all my fault.

CHAPTER 1

———

BELIEVE ME, I WAS NOT looking for a career change when Jack Strawn came to my Emergency Department. It just happened that way. You could say I was primed for it, by an unconscious desire to do something different than medicine, but that would be untrue. If Strawn had not shown up, I would have stayed happy in my job as a sin-city ED physician. After all, I was saving lives and making a good living. Not even a malpractice lawsuit hanging over my head marred my contentment. I even envisioned retiring in my early 50's.

Strawn, age thirty-eight, weighed 394 lbs. and stood 5'9". Super-morbidly obese, BMI of 58. Like others of this body habitus, he showed no neck, a massively protruding abdomen and large ankles with some brawny edema. He came to us around midnight, complaining of a "gout attack." I remember him as very personable, just in a lot of pain from his right big toe.

Las Vegas Memorial Hospital's Emergency Department is a busy place, with two doctors, two physician-assistants and a dozen nurses every shift. We are just off the Strip -- Las Vegas Blvd. -- and our 600 hospital beds and large array of specialists make us the go-to place for local trauma, most Strip ambulance runs and dozens of "walk-ins" daily.

The month was October and I was on the night shift. As you have no doubt heard, "Vegas never sleeps," which means Memorial's ED doesn't slow down much at night. Jack Strawn had a day job as manager of a small apartment building in Summerlin, but other interests brought him to our area at night.

"Let me see that toe."

Strawn sat in a big-boy wheel chair, one of several reserved for the largest patients. He extended his right foot. The toe was twice as large as normal, with some redness below the nail. I touched it lightly and he winced.

"Sorry about that." I turned to the nurse who took his vital signs and chief complaint. Barbara Wilson had been working at Memorial only a few weeks; this was our third shift together. Of medium height, about 130 lbs., she had a pretty face unadorned with very little makeup and nice medium-length wavy brown hair. I remember thinking when I first saw her: *lovely girl, nice body.* After the second shift together, what I really wanted to do was get in bed with Barbara.

All heterosexual men fantasize when they meet a pretty woman, but I thought my fantasy had real possibility. I am only a few years older, in the same profession, and from a good family. Of course being a physician was a big plus. I had not yet asked her out but was getting close. I was hesitant in part because I had a girlfriend of sorts at the time, though she lived in Los Angeles and our relationship was intermittent and probably ending soon. I did not have a girlfriend in Las Vegas and felt a bit lonely.

That Barbara would be *this* patient's nurse on *this* night made me an instant convert to astrology, or whatever those alignments mean when things just happen to come together. *You will meet an unusual person who will facilitate a new love life.*

"Do you have his vital signs?"

Barbara handed me his clipboard and said in a sweet, submissive tone, "Yes, Dr. Luvkin, here they are." She had recently graduated nursing school and was still deferential to doctors. A more experienced nurse would say "Yep, here you go," hand me the clipboard and bop out of the exam room, with "call me if you need anything." But Barbara stood there, in a way I imagine nurses stood by fifty years ago, waiting for the doctor's orders. Lucky for me, since she got to hear my patient's story.

From his brief medical history I learned Mr. Strawn had suffered with gout for about two years, and had "always been heavy because I eat a lot." He was raised in Atlanta and spoke with a southern drawl. He came to us at midnight because "I was in the area and the pain felt real bad." He had run out of his medicine three days earlier and "was too busy to get it renewed."

I ordered some blood tests. "We'll treat it with colchicine," I said, and Barbara quickly retrieved the tablets from a nearby drug cart. She gave him one to swallow, and three more to use until he could get his prescription filled.

I always try to help out my patients with their lifestyle and so asked, "What are you doing about the weight?"

"What do you mean?" Strawn replied.

"It's obviously not healthy. You're only thirty-eight. Quite honestly, you might not make it to fifty with this weight. Have you ever considered bariatric surgery?"

"No, maybe later. I guess I have a few years to go. Hard to lose weight when you eat ten pounds of food a day."

"Wow, that's a lot." I thought of those times when I heard how many pounds of food a bear or elephant eats in a day. I don't remember the numbers, only that with big animals it was always at least two digits. I figure a normal-size human might eat maybe two-three pounds of food a day, if that.

"Well, you need to cut down, begin losing some weight," I said. This recommendation is one of medicine's clichés, so often ignored that -- while true -- it is useless. We say it anyway.

"Hard to do right now. Make money from my weight."

"How's that?" Was he in some sort of carnival act with elephants and bears, to see who could eat the most? Or perhaps on a Las Vegas Sumo wrestling team I knew nothing about? I had never heard of someone making 'money from my weight'. His answer would end up affecting my career at Memorial. Considerably.

"Shittin' contest. I'm one of the best. Can't do it without the food."

I winced and looked at Barbara. This caught Strawn's attention.

"Oh, I'm sorry, Miss," he said, "I shouldn't use that word in mixed company."

"No, that's OK," she replied, in a tone to suggest the patient is always right.

"Let's just call it an elimination contest," Strawn offered. "From front and back."

After two years in Memorial's ED I had seen many bizarre things and nothing really surprised me any longer. Most of the bizarreness was from consensual sexual acts with bad outcomes. A man with a dildo up his rectum, placed so far up we could not extract it in the ED; he went to the operating room for removal. A woman whose uterus suffered a rent from over-aggressive oral sex; she also went to the OR.

We have seen metal rings piercing genitals that led to inflammation or outright infections. And several cases of priapism from using erectile dysfunction drugs. There was one case of coprophagia (eating feces) in a psychiatric patient. I have not yet treated a man with severed penis caused by an angry lover, but have seen one lacerated by teeth marks. And once I saw a guy with a penile rash; he had an allergy to the peanut butter his girlfriend applied so she could lick it off. She came with him and when I offered the diagnosis she calmly said, "Jelly next time."

Strawn's answer intrigued me. What the hell did he mean?

"What do you mean?"

"You eat the food and it comes out the other end, right?"

"Got it," I said.

"Well, the more you eat, the more comes out."

"Makes sense to me." I was happy to play along, hoping of course for some light at the end of Jack's story.

"Well, he who eliminates the most wins the pot. And I win more often than not."

Wow! I thought. *That makes sense. This is Vegas. He who craps the most wins the pot.*

"They weigh it?"

"No, they don't weigh it. They weigh *you*. Before and after. Very clean."

"So it really is an elimination contest," I said.

"Right, just like I said. But those of us who compete, we like to use the s- word."

"And at which casino does this wager take place?" I asked.

"Ain't no casino. It's held at Joe's Plumbing Supplies, over on South Decatur."

I was not familiar with Joe's Plumbing, but it sounded like a legitimate business. "You use their bathroom?"

"He laughed. You never been to Joe's?"

"No, afraid not."

"They got *ten* bathrooms. Each contestant gets his own. Real nice. You got twenty minutes to get rid of your stuff, they you get re-weighed. People watch, people bet. I'm surprised you haven't heard of this. How long you been in Vegas, doc?"

"Is this legal?"

"You mean going to the bathroom? They gonna outlaw that too?"

"No, I mean the betting. Is that controlled by the Gaming Commission?"

"Hell, no. If people want to bet, that's their business. We never been raided, if that's what you mean. Say, you want to come watch one of our contests? We get lots of spectators. You don't have to bet, just come to watch."

"Sure." Why not? I asked myself. It should be interesting.

"OK, give me a piece of paper," he said. "I'll write down the address and date. It ain't gonna be posted on the internet."

I handed him the clip board with a piece of blank paper and he wrote down the date, time and address of Joe's Plumbing Supplies. A quick glance showed the next contest would take place just three days later. When finished, Strawn looked at Barbara and said, "You're invited too, Miss. Lots of women come. We watch our language there."

"Thank you." She blushed a little. At least she didn't recoil in disgust, or reject his invitation outright. I figured she was just being polite.

After Jack Strawn left I took out my phone and googled "Las Vegas elimination contests." I got one of those "disambiguation lists," showing links for boxing, golf, stock car racing and wrestling – popular Vegas sports where *contestants* were eliminated, not their bowels. Then I entered "Las Vegas shitting contest" -- 1.2 million results! All but one entry on the first two web pages was about "Vegas contests" of the more traditional variety. Didn't matter. The first one hit the jackpot, a link to Wikipedia. I clicked on it. The entry was brief, with one of those Wikipedia warnings for sketchy entries: "This article needs additional citations for verification. Please help improve this article by adding citations to reliable sources."

Excretion Contests – Las Vegas
From Wikipedia, the free encyclopedia

Contests whereby men, usually overweight or obese, compete with each other in how much body waste they can excrete over a short, preset time period. The contestant who loses the most body weight wins a pot of money. The money is provided by spectators who place bets – on who they think will win, what the amount of weight loss will be, and other metrics determined at the time of the contest. It is a variation of The Biggest Loser contests popular on television, with the major difference being weight loss is over minutes, not weeks, and comes not from dieting but from bowel elimination.

These contests are known to occur in Las Vegas but have not been confirmed in other cities. Because the betting is not regulated by any agency, and may not conform to all state laws, no web site exists that provides the location or date of the contests;

communication of this information is usually by word of mouth or e-mail. It is not known when these contests began in Las Vegas.

I caught up with Barbara at the nurse's station. Now I had an easy entry. "Look at this," I said, and showed her the Wikipedia text on my cell phone. To my delight, she didn't push me away but read it. Then she looked up at me and smiled, as if to say 'so what'?

"I think I'll go to his next contest," I said, in a casual sort of way, like 'I think I'll go to the next lecture'. To make my decision seem less voyeuristic, I added "professional curiosity, of course." Then I said, oh so casually, to make it sound like I wasn't really asking for a date, "Want to go with me? He said you're invited too."

She looked directly into my eyes but I could not read her emotion. Was she studying my face to see if she liked it? Or was she deciding how to say no without affecting our professional relationship? My heart raced.

"Yes," she said, "it should be interesting."

CHAPTER 2

———◆———

I DID SOME INVESTIGATION. TURNS out Joe's is well known among people in Vegas who shop for plumbing supplies. That meant just about everyone but me. There are three stores in the metro area, and Joe's Plumbing Supplies advertises on TV: "You need it. We got it." The store address Jack provided was three miles west of the hospital on South Decatur, in a strip shopping center. Jack advised arriving before the 10 pm contest time, to get a seat and check out the betting.

The commercial neighborhood could be anywhere USA but for the fact that several stores advertise "Play slots here!" It seemed reassuring that the store fronts were well-lit, and except for the fact that we were looking for a place where they hold elimination contests, nothing seemed out of the ordinary. I did envision getting mugged, with my parents forever commenting: "How could you have been so stupid to go to a plumbing store in the middle of the night? *What* kind of contest?"

"Barbara, are you sure you want to go in?" I asked after we parked.

If she had said no, let's leave, I would have stifled my curiosity and been out of there pronto. But she said, "Sure, we're here, why not?"

We exited the car and walked to Joe's Plumbing. Shades covered the large plate glass windows and a cardboard sign in front said "Store Closed. Private Showing." A heavy guy sat outside in a folding chair, wearing a baseball cap and a flowery, long-sleeved shirt. I wondered if he was one of the contestants.

"What are you looking for?" he asked.

I mumbled something about Jack Strawn inviting us and he opened the door. Pretty informal getting in. It certainly wasn't like the speak-easies of the 1930s, where some guy opens a four x four inch window in a bolted door and asks for a password. I think anyone off the street could have come in. Most likely Joe's door guy just wanted to keep out drunks, kids and anyone who seemed up to no good.

The store was much larger than I imagined from the outside, perhaps 200 feet deep. The front section had been cleared of showroom supplies, and instead held about fifty folding chairs. We got there fifteen minutes early and already the place was dense with people, sitting or milling around. About a third were women.

Two rectangular card-type tables were arranged against one wall. On one table was lemonade and cookies, and copies of the night's "betting sheet." We heard one guy call it by another name that rhymes with betting, which made Barbara wince. Fortunately most of the patrons were not so crude.

A man sat behind another table and before him a short line of people stood waiting to place bets. They gave him cash, he filled out some slip of paper and stuffed the bills in a brown envelope with the contestant's name scribbled on front.

The people were cordial, and Barbara and I struck up conversation with another couple.

"Your first time?" the man asked.

"Yes, it is. How does it work?"

"The betting?"

"Well, yeah, but first, how do they get weighed?"

He pointed to two large scales situated in front of the chairs. "The men will come out, get weighed in boxer shorts, then go to one of Joe's bathrooms. About twenty minutes later they return to get weighed again. Pretty simple."

"And the betting?"

He showed me his sheet. "Lots of ways. You can bet who you think will win in each flight. There's three, based on body weight: between two and three hundred, three to four hundred, and over four hundred pounds. Or, you can bet on the amount of weight to be lost. Whoever gets closest wins that. Or, the order of winners. That gives the greatest odds."

"I see," I replied, "but how did all this get set up? We're new to Vegas and never heard of this before."

"For that you'll have to ask Joe himself. He's over there."

Joe Calabane looked to be about eighty, frail and slightly stooped. I decided not to query the owner and founder. I would get the information elsewhere, later.

"What about women contestants?" Barbara asked.

"No, honey," said the man's wife, "you don't want to go there. Joe's tried it with women a couple of times, but it got a little raucous. You ever see a fat broad in a thin bikini? Guys went nuts. We were there, right George?"

George nodded in agreement and elaborated. "Guys made catcalls, yelled to take their bikinis off, made offers to go sit with them in the bathrooms. One woman freaked out, crapped in front of the audience. Pretty gross. Joe won't deal with women again. Only men."

Within fifteen minutes Barbara and I gained a pretty good idea how things went at these contests. We did not bet, knowing zilch about anyone. The betting sheet showed the three contest flights based on weight, with five names in each. There was no distinction about height or BMI. There were handicapping odds, presumably based on previous wins and other factors unknown to us. Also, we noted only aliases. Jack Strawn's, we learned from asking, was SqueezeHard. Other names I remember were BrownNose, Buttercup, Rosewood and DumpTruck. Real names weren't necessary; these men had *reputations*.

We took a seat in the back, the better to make a quick exit. Could the place be raided? Could we be arrested if the cops showed up? I was thankful we had left no name or email address. At 10 pm the emcee for the evening appeared, a thin man about forty or so, clearly not one of the contestants.

"Ladies and gentlemen," he began, in showmanship fashion, "welcome to tonight's Biggest Loser contests. I trust all of you have placed your bets. After the men are weighed we'll check to see if there are any last minute wagers. The men who will be competing in flight one are, as you can see, behind me." He pointed to a large table about ten yards in back of the scales. Five large men sat in what appeared to be hospital gowns. They were drinking bottled water and eating fruit, in preparation for the contest. Each man wore a cardboard number around his neck: 1, 2, 3, 4 or 5.

"As is our custom, they will get behind one of the screens here, take off their robe and put on fresh, new boxer shorts. This action will be supervised by other contestants and two volunteers from our audience. In this way you will be assured that no contestant is wearing weights or leaded shorts or anything that might increase his body weight. After each contestant has retreated to his private bathroom, you may continue to place bets. Each contestant will have twenty minutes to return and be re-weighed. Any questions?"

A patron in front yelled out: "If a guy wants to get weighed naked, is that allowed?"

"Yes, under the rules, he doesn't have to wear the boxer shorts. The only requirement is the number sign around his neck. Thank you for that question. Any others?"

One by one the men came up, put on the new boxer shorts and got weighed. The process seemed transparent, literally open to inspection if you chose to look. Their weights recorded, the men retreated to the rear bathrooms. At that point two of Joe's minions circulated among the audience, taking more bets. They verbalized each wager to the bettor, then wrote a receipt. "Five point seven pounds." "Number five." "Number three." Barbara and I resisted betting out of sheer ignorance, but were nonetheless fascinated by the activity.

The couple we had spoken with earlier sat next to us.

"Any questions?" the man asked. "Pretty straightforward."

"Who'd you bet on?" I asked.

"Puffnose. Number four. He's our favorite. That guy can dump a lot."

"How much, if I may ask?"

"Just five. Hell, it's worth the price of admission." His wife nodded affirmation.

"And if you win, how much will you get?"

"Three to one odds, fifteen dollars. Minus ten percent for the house."

"The house?"

"Yeah, Joe's house. Right here," and he let out a chuckle.

The winner of Flight One lost 5.7 pounds in the bathroom. Puffnose came in second at 4.3 pounds, so my seatmate was out his five dollars.

Then came round two. More of the same, only heavier guys. Jack Strawn was easily recognized on the far right, contestant number five. He did not recognize us, reason being he didn't really make eye contact with the audience when he was weighed. On his return to the scale he had lost 7.8 lbs. and took first place in his flight. We did not wait for round three and left for the parking lot.

CHAPTER 3

———

IN THE CAR WE HAD the same thought. "What is the attraction?"

"It's the Biggest Loser contest like they have on TV, with a few wrinkles," I said. "There, you diet to lose slowly. Here you eat to lose fast."

"Yes," agreed Barbara, "but the TV show isn't held at Joe's Plumbing. There's a reason for that."

We concluded it was sort of like illegal cockfighting carried out in many parts of the world: a populist approach to flouting authority while engaged in that universal human vice – betting. And like cockfighting, Joe's weight loss contests were grass roots in the extreme, with no chance of being co-opted by any casino. This was the people's betting parlor. We prided ourselves on our analysis and I toyed with the idea of adding text and fresh insight to the Wikipedia article.

Afterwards we went for coffee. I chose Melvin's Diner just off the Strip because it has large booths and is reasonably quiet; you can talk there without raising your voice. In half the restaurants in Las Vegas you almost have to lip read to carry on a conversation.

On the way Barbara and I had discussed little about each other, though I did get her to drop the "doctor" and call me Josh. Seated in a booth at Melvin's, we ordered coffee and a piece of pie to share.

"Excuse me, I've got to go the restroom," said Barbara.

"Me, too."

I washed my hands more thoroughly than usual.

Back in the booth I asked Barbara, "Did you feel dirty after Joe's?"

"A little, but the place itself wasn't actually dirty."

"So, what made you go to nursing school? I assume not right out of high school."

"Hardly. I went to college in Seattle, where I grew up. Majored in English, expecting to be a high school English teacher. Fell in love and got married my senior year."

"You're married?" *Am I wasting my time?*

"Not any more. Lasted two years. He was a graduate student at the time, a great guy I thought. That's a cliché' I suppose, for all the pricks who pose as great guys. He was a jerk, and we parted."

"So that drove you to nursing school?"

"No, it drove me to depression. Plus the fact I couldn't find a teaching job in or near Seattle. Spent all my time substituting. Seems every teacher from kindergarten to twelfth grade has a Masters, or seniority, or a friend in administration. I knew I should go back and get my Masters, but my heart wasn't in it."

I am so afraid of the next question, or rather her answer, but ask it anyway. "Any kids?"

"No. We didn't plan on it right away, and after the first year I realized it wasn't going to work out, and made sure I wouldn't get pregnant." I did not ask how, but wanted to: *Did you use the pill? Did you not sleep with him?*

"So I am having trouble connecting the dots between no teaching job in Seattle and becoming a nurse in Las Vegas. I need a little help here."

"Oh, Josh, it's so obvious." Her sarcasm was sweet, intelligent. "My best girlfriend whom I've known since high school was in Vegas, name's Irene. She's married now but back then she was single. She said I should move here, there were tons of opportunities for a girl with my talent."

"For teaching?"

"No, of course not. For pole dancing."

I was smitten already. She majored in English, recovered from the depression of a failed marriage, moved to Vegas to take up pole dancing, and was now a registered nurse in my ED. What more could I ask for? I just had one question.

"Huh?"

Barbara took a breath, brushed hair away from her forehead and continued. "My girlfriend worked the front desk at The Venetian, and had a second job as pole dancer at the Trader John Saloon. She said the money's great, and you meet all kinds of people."

"I can imagine."

"That's not what lured me here, Josh. Mainly the possibility of starting over, getting far away from my ex and maybe landing a teaching job here. I had no intention of becoming a pole dancer. I didn't even know what it was. So I came and stayed with her for a month, before finding my own place. During that month I went with Irene to Trader John's, to watch her perform."

"And?"

"It's not what you think, or not what I thought. Their clientele includes a lot of couples, not just dirty old men, and every evening they invite women from the audience to perform. Their husbands or boyfriends think it's a hoot."

"Sorry," I said, "but what is *it*? For those of us from the Midwest, sounds like the first step toward sex for money. What we in old-fashioned land call the big P."

"I know, I know. But in the higher class places, that's not apparent. Believe it or not, they will kick out any customer who tries to hit on the girls, fondle or proposition them. It's one hundred percent looky-no touchy."

Our order arrived and we each took a bite of Melvin's delicious peanut butter chocolate pie.

"So where's the money come in? Girls don't do it for peanuts. If they did, I could see monkeys in that gig."

She did not laugh. Sometimes my jokes fall flat.

"You show your butt off, your boobs, one at a time, rarely if so inclined your crotch. Men throw money at you. You scoop it up."

"Is this the same as lap dancing?

"Hardly. They have that too, but that's more touchy-feely. Some girls go for that, but pole dancing is more of an art form. It's just you and a pole."

"Literally, a pole?"

"Literally, a pole. About this big around." She curved her thumb and index finger to show about three inches in diameter. "Goes from floor to ceiling."

"How did you know what to do with the pole?"

"Took a few lessons."

"Really? Some girls flunk?"

"No one flunks. Once they let you take the lessons you've more or less passed."

"You mean you've slept with the boss."

"Boy, you are cynical. It just means you've auditioned in a bikini."

She enjoyed the bantering and could take any question I asked. Each minute in that booth I grew more attracted to her.

"Something's not connecting here, Barbara, if I may be so blunt. You come from Seattle, recently divorced, hoping to be a school teacher. And within a month or so of being in Vegas you are auditioning for pole dancing?"

"Insane, isn't it?"

"I'll say."

"The truth is, I have the right figure and the money offered was more than I could make as a teacher. I felt confident from Irene that this was legitimate and nothing would be expected of me for sexual favors. I mean there's a pole dancer's union, for God sakes. So I tried it one night, enjoyed myself, and went on from there."

"So naturally this led to nursing."

"Of course."

"You're teasing me now, Barbara. How did you get from the dancing pole to the IV pole?"

"I did it for about a year. The novelty wore off. There were a couple of assholes who were a little frightening, but they were quickly bounced. So while the money was good, for not a whole lot of work, I saw there was no future." She fondled her coffee cup in both hands, and I envisioned her fondling something else.

"Well, I agree with that," I said.

"I began making inquiries about getting my Masters in education. Thought of going to UNLV, or doing it online through the University of Phoenix, or even moving to another city, though I really liked Vegas. But as I read about all the career opportunities, most of the jobs were for medicine, nursing, medical techs. Not so much for education, even with a Masters. I made a career change, almost instantly.

"So from teaching to nursing, in an instant. That's impressive."

"I wanted a career with a decent income, one where I can help people. I was accepted to UNLV's nursing school and three years later had my RN. Right away got the job at Memorial. It's really that simple."

I took another bite of pie. "How old are you, if I may ask?"

"You may ask. Twenty-seven. Getting up there. And you?"

"Thirty-three. Do you still pole dance?"

"I was afraid you were going to ask. I did it through nursing school, about once a week. That's how I paid for school, along with loans and some help from my parents. Now I'm going to quit. Soon."

"You don't sound so sure." She smiled, as I if had found out a deep secret.

"I'm sure, just not sure when. I can still make as much in two hours some nights as on a twelve-hour nursing shift."

I was going to ask about "relationships" since her move to Vegas, but she changed the subject.

"Enough about me," she said. "Tell me about yourself."

I am superb at taking a history – it's part of evaluating patients – but not so much at giving one. I did not want to bore her and just gave a telescoped summary. Grew up in Cleveland, Dad's an orthopedic surgeon,

Mom's an OR nurse, older sister is a pediatrician with two kids. Parents wanted me to go to medical school, but I majored in liberal arts and playing the guitar. Wasn't attracted to medicine. After college spent several months in India. Then in Delhi one night decided I would, after all, go into medicine.

"Slow down, I'm dizzy," she said. "How did you end up in India?"

"So you don't like the Readers' Digest history?"

"Readers' Digest? You're more like the Twitter version."

This was good. She *was* interested.

"Did I mention Wendy?"

"She's your sister?"

"No, the girl I went to India with."

"I think you're having a little expressive aphasia right now. Not very coherent."

"Sorry, guess I'm just so afraid of boring you."

"So you mention an old girl friend? That's supposed to interest me?"

"She's why I went to India."

"So you're just giving me teasers about your past. Do you want me to ask twenty questions?"

"Go ahead."

"Did you marry Wendy?"

"No."

"Did you sleep with Wendy?"

"Yes."

"Then what happened?"

"OK, I'm sorry, twenty questions won't do it. I'll tell you more, just promise to cut me off when it gets boring."

"Don't worry, I will."

"So in high school I had learned to play guitar reasonably well, even tried composing a couple of songs. When I got to college I met other like-minded wannabe Bob Dylans."

"You mean guys who write poetry but can't sing?"

"Well, yeah, if you want to look at it that way. There was a jam session almost every night in local coffee houses, and I learned most of the songs by heart. I took one science course, Biology, and got a B. Every time I went home Mom and Dad would ask, "Are you going to apply to medical school? What are you going to do with your life?" My answer was always the same. "Right now I'm learning a lot about the world." They thought it was BS, but that would back them off for a while."

"OK," Barbara said. I can relate to that. I was in liberal arts before I found nursing."

"Anyway, between my junior and senior year of college I worked at Yellowstone, at Old Faithful Inn, right across from the famous geyser. Ever been there?"

"No, it's on my list. I've been to Bryce and Zion, though."

"Yeah, me too. Magnificent. Anyway, those park lodge jobs tend to be menial but not easy to come by, so I was glad to get it. I cleaned rooms, worked as a waiter and busboy, did some lodge maintenance, all for the privilege of spending eight weeks in God's Country."

She looked at me doe-eyed. I was capturing her imagination and she was not bored. "On days off I hiked and got to visit most of the tourist sites. One in particular is called Artist's Point, which overlooks The Grand Canyon of the Yellowstone. It's an amazing vista. Let me show it to you." I pulled out my cell phone, googled the site and in less than a minute had a picture.

"Wow," she said. "Sort of reminds me of the canyon in Zion, except for the waterfall."

"Yeah, well it's even more impressive in person."

"So this is where you met Wendy?"

"Actually, yes. We had a thing going at Yellowstone. She was sort of hippie-like, and told me she was going to India after her college graduation in California. Her plan was to study at an ashram and she asked me to join her. I said yes, since I had no better plans after graduation. It seemed like a cool thing to do."

"And let me guess," said Barbara. "Your parents weren't happy."

"That's an understatement. They went ballistic, but in the end they really had no choice. I was prepared to pay my own way with savings from the summer job. That money would have run out in a few months. My father was afraid I'd end up destitute and sick in India. He agreed to fund the trip if I promised to take pre-med when I returned and consider medical school. That's a condensed version of a bitter struggle that lasted the better part of a week."

The waitress brought the check, and pointedly asked if we wanted anything else. The place was busy and I got the feeling she wanted the booth for new customers. I gave her my credit card.

"So please continue," Barbara said. "This is interesting."

"So do you know what an ashram is?"

"Sort of. A place of meditation. Guru and all."

"Exactly. Wendy found our ashram through a friend in California who had studied in India. It was located five miles outside Nagpur, a city south of Delhi. The ashram specialized in young Americans who wanted to 'find their way'. That sort of fit us."

"Not the Ritz Carlton, I take it."

"Hardly. For my taste it was downright Spartan. A couple of low slung buildings built of stucco, with mattresses on the floor for sleeping. Mostly vegetarian food, mostly no toilets or hot showers, and mostly meditation and study during the day, kind of boring. But there were two huge plusses."

"Wendy being one," she said. "What's the other?"

"Music. I was pleasantly surprised about the music. It was authentic Indian music. Do you play an instrument?"

"No, not really, but I used to sing in a choir."

"Well, Indian music is on a different scale system than in the west. The sitar is a distant cousin to our stringed instruments. It opened my eyes to Eastern melodies and intervals. Native Hindis played it in the evenings, and when I brought out my guitar to perform, they listened politely. My Western-style folk songs sounded strange to them, but as music is the universal language there was mutual appreciation."

"So a jam session, Indian style."

"Sort of. Actually, the majority of the ashram visitors were from the states, so they joined in singalongs that reminded them of home. We played *The Sloop John B.* and *This Land Is Your Land* and a bunch of other American folk songs. The music opportunities were good, an unexpected bonus."

"But you broke up with Wendy?"

"Well, that's a short story. Want to hear it?"

"I'm all ears."

"Probably the only real requirement to survive in the Nagpur ashram was that you not disturb the peace. Our visit brought in needed income. I think we each paid about $200 a month to stay there. The head guru was one Dittyram Suburambian, who looked to be about sixty. His English was not very good but he understood American money, so we got alone fine."

"So let me guess. This Dittyram guy falls in love with Wendy and you lose her to his higher spirituality."

"Close. Not bad. You see, all along Wendy's goal was to quote find myself unquote. My goals were somewhat more prosaic. I remember making a list. Have sex with her. Learn about the culture of another country. Avoid my parents for a reasonable period. And decide what to do with my next fifty years or so. I succeeded on all counts but one."

"I can imagine which one. You learned about India. You avoided your parents. You have a long medical career ahead of you. That leaves…"

"Yeah, well, the more Wendy prayed, studied and meditated, the less inclined she was to sleep with me. Actually, there was communal sleeping, so there was no privacy at night. We had to go off a ways to do it, which was not that difficult. In any case, the teachings of this ashram did not exactly conform to my idea of sex. Do you know what she told me?"

"Something spiritual, I'm sure."

"Say, you're good. She said, "Josh, we must love the spirit more than the body." Can you believe that?"

"I mean you went with her to the ashram. Did you think it was going to be Club Med?"

"Who the hell knows? All I know is she was brainwashed. I was blunt. I told her "Yes, but I need you." And she said…?"

"You want me to guess?"

"Go ahead. You've nailed her pretty good so far."

"OK, she said, 'Yes, Josh, but the needs are spiritual, not physical'."

"Dead on! That's exactly what she said! Do you know Wendy?"

"She's my sister."

For a half-second I believed her, but then she put a hand around my forearm and looked at me with twinkly eyes. "Oh, I'm just joshing with you, Josh. The way you tell this, her responses seem obvious. As you said, she was brainwashed."

"Yeah, well, it was a deal breaker, that's for sure. By the end of the first month sex was down to less once a week, and then with an embellishment. Guess again."

"She had the guru right there, praying for your soul."

"OK, good guess, but a little off this time. *She* prayed during the act, like she was screwing some god and not me. By the end of two months we were done. I left after the third month, and toured India with a guy I met in the ashram."

Just then the waitress brought over the credit card receipt, which I signed. "I think they want us out of here, to make room for other customers."

"Well, you have to tell me what happened with Wendy."

"God knows," I said. "About the time we broke up she became the close companion of the Guru's assistant, a young Hindi named Swami Gupta. I suspected she was doing it with him. Or doing *something* with him to give her the same kick as sex with me. I left her in India. That was twelve years ago. She's probably a Maharani by now."

Barbara laughed, a totally guileless laugh that made me feel I had conquered her soul. *She likes me.* I could have regaled her for another hour about my past. Seeing her genuine interest, however, I did suggest she and I were two like-minded vagabonds, each seeking a new beginning in Las Vegas.

"Seems that way," she agreed.

I would use the promise of *more Josh history* for another date. "India was fascinating, but I think it's best for another time."

Barbara pouted with her lips in a way to suggest she wanted more history – or just didn't want the date to end so soon. My thought as well. That night I discovered someone special: a woman with beauty, brains, determination and charm. I wanted her in my bed more than ever. I looked at my watch. An hour had gone by since we sat down and it was past midnight.

"Well, this has been fun."

"Yes, it has."

"I'll take you home" I said, which is not what I wanted to do. I decided to be bold. "Unless you want to come to my place. I live close by, in the Abington Tower." She knew what I meant, of course. *Unless you want to sleep with me tonight.*

"I don't know. Do you have a pole in your apartment?"

CHAPTER 4

———

ON THE DRIVE TO MY apartment she told me her ex was a jerk but a lover, and never physically abused her. The abuse was all emotional. He played around. I casually asked if she was seeing anyone else and she said no. She asked me the same, and I admitted to dating a woman who lived in Los Angeles, but said the relationship was over. In my mind it was; I just did not tell Barbara that Judy had not yet received official notice.

We joked about coming together because some morbidly obese guy told me he liked to bet on...well, I've explained all that.

I could not believe my luck. We each had a physical and emotional need at that point in our lives, and clicked on every level. And Barbara was glorious in bed. That she had been married did not hurt in the experience department. Fortunately we were both off work the next day and could sleep in. My plan was to take her home in the morning, but she would stay the night. After we made love it was blissful to just lie next to her with gentle caresses and fall asleep in her arms.

The bliss ended abruptly around 3 am when she nudged me awake. "Are you up?"

"Yeah, what's the matter?"

"I think someone's here," she whispered. "I heard a door open. There's a light on in the living room." I could tell she was frightened and held her close.

"Shhh. Don't say anything."

My one-bedroom apartment is on the 15th floor of a luxury tower, with a doorman round the clock. How would an intruder get in? The bedroom door was half-open and I affirmed Barbara's observation. The light was on *and* there was someone in the living room. There was some rustling, like a coat coming off.

I did not blame Barbara for thinking we were being burglarized. It was instinct to be frightened. Was I scared? Actually, no. After coming to my senses I was pretty sure who it was.

"Stay here. I'll check it out," I whispered.

"Be careful."

"Don't worry."

I went into the living room and closed the bedroom door behind me. Next to the couch stood Judy Berkowitz. She had a small valise, set down on the coach near where she stood.

"Judy, what are you doing here?"

"I called you on your cell phone and left a message."

"Oh, I didn't check it."

"Remember last week, I said I might come in? Well, I made it. You look surprised. Is something wrong?"

"No, no, not at all, I just didn't know you were coming, that's all."

"Well, aren't you glad to see me?"

I walked over and put my arms lightly on her shoulders, as you might when meeting an old friend. Mainly I didn't want Judy to go into the bedroom. She nudged against me and positioned herself for a kiss. I could not refuse.

"Josh, you seem distant. What's the matter? I'm so tired. I need to lie down."

The bedroom door opened and Barbara walked in, wearing only my shirt from last night. She was otherwise naked and her thighs glistened in the light. *This is not good.*

Our lips had just had just parted but I still had my arms around the intruder.

"Who's that?" Barbara asked.

I moved back a step. "Barbara, this is Judy."

"Who is Judy?"

Judy stared at this unexpected woman, then at me, then back at Barbara. "Who is Judy? Who is Judy? I'm his wife, honey."

"Oh?"

"Who the hell are you?" asked Judy.

I felt like I was in a sitcom, which was a strange thought because it wasn't so funny. I remember wishing I was a thousand miles away. I turned to Barbara and blurted: "She is *not* my wife. She's the woman I mentioned to you who I was dating in LA. I mean from LA. She has a key to the apartment, and came in tonight. I didn't know she was coming. That's it. No secrets. It's just unfortunate, uh, timing."

"Not his wife?" rejoined Judy. "Barbara dear, look in the second from the top drawer of his dresser. There you will find panties and bras, if he hasn't thrown them out. Either your boyfriend is a cross dresser or he's living with another woman. Who happens to be me!"

"Judy, why are you telling her we're married?" I couldn't deny we were living together, given the physical evidence, though technically we were not. But the marriage lie was too much. I thought of asking Judy, *if we're married where's your wedding ring?* but decided against it. She might respond that the stone was being re-set, or some other such fabrication. It would become a he-said-she-said situation, one I could not win at that particular moment.

"Why are you sleeping with a whore?" Judy retorted. Get on her wrong side and Judy can bite. At that moment I had a vision of Glenn Close in *Fatal Attraction*.

Barbara disappeared into the bedroom and returned a minute later with a handful of panties and bras. "Josh, *are* you a cross dresser?"

It was over in five minutes. Barbara dressed and stormed out of the apartment. She would not let me take her home, said she would call a cab. On the way out she had the last word, and it was a doozy: "If you ever divorce the bitch, let me know," and with that slammed the door.

Judy is an ED doctor like me. I knew her from medical school. She married a guy in our class, and went to LA to do a residency in Emergency Medicine while he trained in general surgery. The marriage lasted but two years -- ironically, same as Barbara's. I met Judy again at a Vegas convention for ED physicians, learned she was single again. She is Jewish, as am I, which gave her one point on the Josh Luvkin date-ability scale. Being a doctor gave her another point. And, to tell the truth, she is attractive, bosomy and sexually experienced – two more points. Finally, she was looking for a man she could trust for sex, which figured for six points. Bingo!

One thing led to another, and for several months we had been commuting to each other's homes to screw whenever our schedules allowed. But all those points couldn't counteract the fact that she had become controlling and demanding in an uncomfortable way. I felt confined when around her, as if I was being graded on my words and actions. The sex was good but the after-sex, not so much.

She told me her ex-husband had been more in love with the hospital than with her – he was there night and day – and blamed him for the breakup. I wondered if he just found her impossible to live with. They parted amiably, she said.

After six months of back and forth dating, Judy hinted strongly that she would like to move to Vegas and get married. She sort of assumed, because of all the points, that I would want that as well. "Won't your parents be happy if you married a Jewish doctor?" she said, only half in jest. *But would I be happy?* The deep down answer was no. Since we lived 200 miles apart, and I was largely free from her everyday clutches, I merely put her off rather than cut her off. After finding Barbara I was definitely going to end the relationship, but she showed up before I had the chance.

Now Judy was horny and wanted to screw.

"I just drove four hours, Josh. I'm tired and just want to get in bed with you. I really don't care about Barbara. Forget about her. I need you."

"I can't," I said. "I just did it and there's nothing there."

"I'll take care of that" she said, rolling her tongue.

Again *Fatal Attraction* popped into my head. I did not want to become rabbit stew. I swore this would be the last time.

———————

Satisfying Judy's lust improved her demeanor. Afterwards, lying in bed, she was somewhat apologetic.

"I'm sorry I called your friend a whore. But what did you expect after I come home and find her in our bed?"

"Your home is in Los Angeles."

"You know what I mean. My Las Vegas home."

"Why did you have to say we're married? That really scared her off."

"How long have you been dating her?"

"This was the first time."

"Wow, we didn't even do it the first date."

"Actually, we did."

"Whatever. Do you plan to continue fucking her while I'm in LA?"

"Judy, can we discuss this in the morning? It was my first date with her and I don't know what I'm going to do. I wish you hadn't said we were married."

"It just came to me. It's almost like we're married, considering my clothes are here and I have a key."

At that point I knew I had to extricate myself. However, I also had to go back to sleep, and didn't want to worry about waking with a genital injury. Which I envisioned if I broke off the relationship at that moment.

"That's true, so it makes sense, Judy. Let's get some sleep, OK?" I hugged her to show my affection, as if nothing had changed.

"OK," she said, and we fell asleep.

After waking, we showered, dressed, and sat down for breakfast in my small kitchen off the living room. So far there had been no mention of the night before. Now safely seated, I was determined to end our relationship fully clothed, my genitals safely inside jockey shorts and long pants.

"Judy, can we discuss last night?"

"What's to discuss? You had a bitch in bed with you, you're unfaithful. Don't do it again."

I decided on a bold approach. "I like her, Judy."

"She's a slut."

"She's not a slut. She's a nice girl, and she lives here in Vegas and it's not really working out well with me and you."

Judy stared at me. Here is where the hack writer inserts *If looks could kill*....

"*What* are you saying?"

"Look, Judy, you know I like you, and we've had some great times together, but I'm not ready for marriage. I like this new girl a lot and in all fairness it's just better if we stop seeing each other. I'm just being honest."

"You're serious, aren't you?"

"Yes, can't this be our last time? No hard feelings?" The way I approached this must seem strange, like I'm asking permission to end the relationship. But I couldn't get *Fatal Attraction* out of my head.

"When do you want me to leave?"

"Well, if you feel like driving back to LA, I guess today. I see you didn't bring a suitcase, just that little valise. I'll give you one of mine, you can pack your clothes. Keep the suitcase. But no point in prolonging this. It's painful for both of us. Is that OK?"

"I don't want the fucking clothes! I have no more room in my closets. Give them to Barbara." They would not fit Barbara, who is taller and thinner, but I didn't belabor the point.

"OK, it's up to you. The suitcase is yours if you want to pack."

"So you're going to kick me out?"

"No, Judy, I'm not kicking you out. You want to stay longer? Fine. I'm just saying, I think the relationship is over for now." Don't know why I said "for now." Fortunately she didn't ask for an interpretation.

"So, it's like I'm being fired. You're going to walk me to the front door?"

"Whatever you want," I said. "I'm going to continue dating Barbara, if she'll have me back after last night."

"So this is it for us?"

"Yes, I'm afraid so."

She started to cry. I felt badly, and came over to her. She pushed me away. Thankfully, she was not vicious, just sad. Pathetic even.

"I'll go. You won't be bothered by Judy Berkowitz again."

"Can't we stay friends? I'll see you at med school reunions."

"Sure." She held out her hand. I pulled her toward me and hugged her.

"No hard feelings?"

"I'll be fine," she said. "I'm OK."

"Maybe I'll also see you at another ED convention," I said. "They always seem to be in Vegas."

"Yeah, sure. Let me go to the bathroom and freshen up, then I'll leave."

Is she going to kill herself? Isn't that what happens in novels? Or, is she going to pull out a small gun hidden in her purse, and kill me? I really wanted her out of the apartment. I prayed she would go peacefully.

"Of course," I said, "whatever you have to do."

She went into the bathroom and came out a few minutes later. "You want to walk me to the car?"

"Is it in the garage?"

"Yes." I was afraid to ask her for the apartment key she had used to gain entry the night before. I decided I would change the lock on the apartment. To my surprise, she offered up the key.

"I have the apartment key. Here it is," and she handed it over. "I suppose you'll want to give it to Barbara." I did not reply. We took the elevator to the basement, found her car, a Prius hybrid. I didn't ask for the garage swipe card, an extra one I had secured for her when she first came to Vegas. By this point I felt more than a little guilty, but made a mental note to change my own parking spot, in case she returned looking for my car. Then I repeated, "Judy, I do want to stay friends, OK?"

"Sure, sure." I put her valise in the trunk and she got in the driver's seat.

"If you need anything I can help with, obviously call me, OK?"

"OK," she said, and pulled out of the parking spot. I watched as she turned left at the garage exit sign, heaved a sigh of relief and returned to my apartment. I checked my watch - 9:15 am.

———◆———

I waited until 10 o'clock before calling Barbara. She could not have fallen asleep until 4 am. Her cell phone announced the caller.

"Hello Josh." At least she answered, a good sign.

"I'm really sorry about last night. The good news is she's gone. Forever."

"Are you filing for divorce?"

"Barbara, we're not married. Never were. Judy's just a little nutso."

"OK, I understand. No actually, I don't understand. I'm a little upset. I sleep with you on our first date, and then your other girlfriend who, you remember, you told me you were through with, enters your apartment and says she lives there. What do you expect me to think?"

I was feeling desperate. I did not want to lose Barbara.

"You're right, it was insane. In my mind I was done with her, but not in her mind. I was going to call her today and tell her we were done, but she just showed up. I have nothing to hide. Can we meet for lunch? I really want to see you again."

"Can't today. Have some errands to run."

"Dinner?"

"Look, Josh, I'm still a little shaken by last night. I've never been called a whore before. Let's just cool it for a while, give me some time to think. Is that reasonable? I had one bad relationship and don't need another."

Ouch! I realized any further pressure would just backfire.

"No, of course I understand. I really do. When is your next shift at Memorial?"

"Tomorrow night."

"Mine too," I said. "I guess I'll see you then. I just have one thing to say, Barbara."

"What's that?"

"I love you."

———◆———

Unlike most medical specialties, emergency medicine gives you a lot of time off. The work is so intense for a single twelve-hour shift, you need the time to recuperate. Typically, ED doctors work no more than four shifts a week before taking a sizable break. Schedules vary all over the place; sometimes we do four shifts in in a row, followed by three or four days off. Sometimes we work every other day for two weeks, then have several days off.

On my off days I have lots to do. I may go shopping, hike at Red Rock Canyon or practice my guitar. I will also check out the latest casino, but only for its ambience, décor and restaurants; I don't waste time at the tables or slot machines.

Since Barbara was not meeting me for lunch I decided to go shopping. I wanted a new guitar and had my eye on a Martin D17M model at Sam Ash Music. The Las Vegas franchise is a great store; you can spend an hour or more trying out various instruments, and if you don't like the stock model they'll special order one for you. After almost ninety minutes in the store – relaxation time for me – I came home with the new Martin.

At first I thought it was the wrong apartment. The place was trashed. Broken dishes on the floor, couch pillows in the bathtub, dresser drawer contents strewn about the bed, lamps upended. Bathroom toiletries littered the tile floor, some of the bottles opened; there was goo and gel in puddles. It looked like a tornado had invaded every room. But the windows were not broken and I detected nothing amiss with the front door lock.

My apartment had been burglarized, no doubt, but it was not obvious what, if anything, was missing. Fortunately, except for my passport and family photos, I had nothing that couldn't easily be replaced. The TV, my old guitar and a small trove of rare medical books I collect were still in place. What could the burglar have been looking for? I hated the thought of cleaning up. First, though, I would report the burglary to the super's office; maybe he had information on other break-ins. As I was about to leave my eye caught red lettering at the top of the fridge door, evidently written in lipstick.

"Forgot a pair of shoes I wanted, so came back for them. Have a nice day. JB."

CHAPTER 5

———◆———

THE NEXT NIGHT VICKI LEDBETTER, a pretty 24-year-old woman on her honeymoon at The Venetian, came to the ED with complaint of "my asthma is acting up." Her husband of just five days brought her in by cab. Ambulance runs get priority, so neither I nor the other physician saw her immediately. The triage nurse put Vickie in a room and Barbara was assigned to take vital signs.

The shift was only an hour old and we had not said more than a few words to each other, and those few were all in the line of work. Barbara did not appear angry or vengeful, just distant. My plan was to approach her after the shift, to see when we might get together, if only for coffee and to talk things over.

An aide came to my side. "You are needed in room eight, Dr. Luvkin. Miss Wilson said to come right away." I walked over quickly.

As I opened the curtain Barbara turned and spoke. "Dr. Luvkin, I think you should see this new patient, Mrs. Ledbetter. Her peak flow is only ninety." Peak flow is a measurement of asthma severity, obtained after a patient blows into a tube. Less than 150 in an adult is a pretty bad attack.

Mr. Ledbetter, about the same age as his wife, was at her side. She was using her neck muscles to help in breathing, which is always ominous: a sign of working hard to get air into her lungs. She sucked on a nebulizer to inhale albuterol, standard initial treatment for an asthma attack. Before even listening to her chest I asked Barbara if she had received any steroids.

"Not yet."

"Let's give her 125 SoluMedrol, IV push." Barbara went for the medication.

"When did this begin?"

"Couple of hours ago," her husband offered. "There was smoking in the casino, and she'd been having a cold the past couple of days. So I guess the combination."

"She doesn't smoke, I assume."

"No. Me neither."

"History of asthma?

The patient nodded yes.

I didn't want her to stop inhaling the albuterol, but needed a little more information. "Ever had an attack like this one?"

She nodded yes.

I looked at the clip board. Intake history read: "Hx asthma 5 years. Attack began @1900. Allergic to pollen, ragweed. Takes Symbicort, ProAir. Prn prednisone x2/year. On BCP. Smoking (-). Married 5 d. ago. On h-moon at Venetian."

"Ever had to be hospitalized for asthma before?"

She nodded yes and held up two fingers.

"Twice?"

She nodded. Her husband squeezed her hand. "You'll be fine, honey. Just hang in there," he said.

I listened to her chest and heard faint, distant wheezing. Heart rate 140. Respirations 35. All bad signs.

Barbara arrived with the SoluMedrol and pushed 125 mg into Vicki's IV.

"Barbara, let's give her another albuterol treatment when this one's finished, and then re-check the peak flow. "

I wanted to make Vicki feel less anxious, and tried a little casual conversation with her husband. "Newly married, huh?"

"Yes, five days," he said.

"Where are you from?"

"Chicago."

"First time in Vegas?" I conversed with him but my eyes were on his wife. So far, no sign of improvement. Her neck muscles bobbed up and down.

"My second time, her first. You think she'll be OK, doc?"

"Well, she's got some powerful medicine on board. She certainly won't leave here until we're sure she's stable."

Barbara would stay in the room until relieved or Vicki was out of danger. I went to see another patient, a 65-year alcoholic who fell off a slot machine stool at Mandalay Bay. He was drunk and complained of chest wall pain. I ordered x-rays to make sure there were no rib fractures or pneumothorax. As I finished with him the same nurse's aide came to get me. "Miss Wilson needs you, Dr. Luvkin."

"OK, come with me." We went right over.

"Peak flow's only 70, Josh." At least she used my first name this time.

"OK, let's get a stat blood gas." The aide left to get the respiratory tech.

"What's going on, Doctor?" Mr. Ledbetter asked. She was not improving, the situation increasingly serious by the minute. There was real risk of exhaustion setting in. Then she would quit breathing. I asked him to step outside the room so we could talk. Barbara remained with the patient.

"She's working very hard to breathe," I explained. "I'm afraid she's tiring out."

"So she's getting worse?"

"Her asthma is not responding, at least not quickly enough," I explained. "Has she ever been on life support for this problem, to your knowledge?"

His eyes widened. "I don't get what you mean."

"Do you know if your wife has ever been in the intensive care unit, for her asthma?"

"Not to my knowledge. This is really bad, isn't it?"

"Seems so," I replied. "I don't want to alarm you, but we may need to put a tube in her throat and put her on a breathing machine until her asthma resolves. It's very severe. I would like to ask you to stay outside until we make this decision. You can stay right here. Give me a few minutes."

I returned to her bedside. Respiratory Therapy was there, drawing the arterial blood gas. They got it on the first try, from her radial artery. It only took a couple of minutes to get the results. I put my stethoscope to her chest. Now I could hardly hear any air movement.

The tech returned with the ABG results: pH 7.25, PCO2 61, PO2 75 (on oxygen). The numbers indicated acute respiratory failure and high likelihood of dying without mechanical ventilation.

"Barbara, get the cart. And get Dr. Munson, please." If the other physician is not tied up in a dire emergency, our policy for emergency intubations is to have both ED physicians in the room.

The crash cart and my shift colleague Bill Munson arrived seconds later.

"What's going on?" Bill asked. I gave him a quick synopsis. He would stand by to offer any needed assistance. I turned to the patient.

"Vicki, your breathing is not improving. I'm going to put a tube in your throat so we can take over the breathing for you. I explained this to your husband and he understands." She was hardly able to respond. She was about to go out on me.

"Propofol, 100 micrograms push, then run a drip."

The order was carried out swiftly.

We lowered her bed to the supine position and the respiratory therapist began bagging her with an Ambu bag attached to a face mask. Each push of the bag would force enough air into Vicki's lungs to keep her alive until the tube was placed. Once the tube was placed, the mechanical ventilator would take over.

"She's very tight, Dr. Luvkin,"

"I know. Make sure she's getting 100% oxygen. What's her O2 sat?"

"Ninety-two percent."

"Good."

I stood behind my patient and asked the Ambu bagger to stop giving Vickie breaths. I opened Vicki's mouth as wide as possible. She was now sedated. I placed the lighted intubation blade in her mouth, depressed the tongue and began searching for vocal cords.

"Suction."

She fought a little. I was afraid to paralyze her, since then all breathing effort would cease; if the tube didn't get placed properly she could die quickly.

"Another 100 of Propofol, please, as fast as you can get it in. Keep bagging."

Two minutes later I was ready to try again.

"OK, I'm above the cords. Barbara please press gently on her neck." I could see the vocal cords indent slightly from Barbara's pressing. I was clearly in the right place. I pushed the clear plastic endotracheal tube down her throat and through the open cords.

"It's through. Get an end tidal, please."

The respiratory therapist attached the end tidal PCO_2 monitor between the end of the endotracheal tube and ventilator circuit. The monitor changed colors, signifying proper exhalation of CO_2. The tube was where it was supposed to be, in her trachea.

"OK, keep her on 100% oxygen, tidal volume 500, rate 14. And please order a chest x-ray." These cryptic orders were fully understood by Barbara and the respiratory therapist.

"What's her sat now?" I asked.

"Ninety-eight percent."

"Excellent."

"Need me anymore?" Bill asked.

"No, thanks Bill. I'll stay with her until she gets upstairs."

With all the orders in place, I stepped into the hallway and approached Mr. Ledbetter. He was sitting in a chair.

"We had to put the tube in her throat. She's stable for now, but on life support. She'll go to the ICU, and other doctors will take over her care."

"Will she, will she…?"

"She should do OK, unless there is some unexpected catastrophe. She's young and appears otherwise healthy. That's in her favor." I wanted to be optimistic, but not make any promises. "We have treated many patients like your wife, so this is reversible. You did the right thing bringing her here when you did."

"How long will she be on life support?"

"I really can't predict. As short as a day, as long as a week. All this will be easier to determine after the first twenty-four hours. For now, she'll go to the ICU."

I returned to Vickie's room, reassured by the gentle whoosh of the ventilator and my patient's oxygen saturation: 100%.

Ten minutes later I had the ICU team down to get their patient. Vicki was lucky, and we were lucky. If felt good to be a physician.

I did not have to wait until the end of the shift. About an hour later, during a quiet period, Barbara came up to me.

"Don't let it go to your head Josh, but I was very impressed with what you did."

I tried to be modest. "Thanks, but that's my job."

"I know, but I'm new at this, remember. I haven't seen emergency intubation before. And it's only the second time I've given Propofol. The first time was a GI procedure, nothing like this. You saved her life."

"I hope so. Does this mean you'll go out with me again?"

"Are you asking?"

"What do you think? Coffee after work?"

"That would be nice," she said.

"And if Mrs. Ledbetter had died?" I asked.

Barbara just smiled and didn't answer. I didn't press her, either.

After work we went to Melvin's Diner and talked for a good hour. I told her Judy was gone from my life, and explained how I personally escorted her to the garage. Barbara didn't ask why Judy had spent the night. I hoped she assumed it was not inappropriate, given the lateness of the hour.

I did not tell her about Judy's unexpected return to my apartment, or how she trashed it, or the fact that she must have made copies of the door key. I also omitted my changing of the lock and adding an inside dead bolt. Not telling her any of this, I also didn't have to explain my decision not to report the incident. I would tell her these things, but not now, not when I was desperate to re-establish our relationship.

"Barbara, do you remember what I said the other day, on the phone?"

"About you not being married?

"No, about my feelings toward you."

"No, don't remember. Remind me."

I mouthed the words.

"Oh, yes, now I remember. Well, I've heard that before, you know."

"You know what they say on Wall Street?" I asked.

"There's a sucker born every minute?"

"No, not that one. The other saying. 'It's different this time'. Will you move in with me?"

She did not seem surprised by the question, but didn't answer right away either.

I raised my eyebrows and opened my palms.

"I'm thinking," she said.

CHAPTER 6

———

SHE MOVED IN. WE ARRANGED our work schedules to coincide as much as possible, so we could be off at the same times.

A week after we got back together, I heard Barbara singing in one of the ED rooms. I pulled back the curtain and saw her wrapping a bandage around the arm of a three-year old boy. The boy's mother was holding his other arm. As she wrapped, she sang.

> Ah unk! went the little green frog one day.
> Ah unk! went the little green frog.
> Ah unk! went the little green frog one day.
> and we all go Ah unk! Unk! Unk!

Every time Barbara said Ah unk! she rushed at the boy's face with a big smile, then retreated with "went the little green frog." Each time the boy laughed, and his mother too. *She's marvelous with the child.* Right then I wanted to hug and kiss her.

Barbara turned to me. "Oh, hi Dr. Luvkin. This is Timothy. He had a little accident." I picked up the ED sheet. Laceration of left arm from a fall. The plastic surgeon had just left.

"Wow, ten stitches, I said. Doesn't he get a lollipop? Where are the lollipops?" Mom stroked his forehead.

Timothy said "Lollipop!"

I went to find the candy. On my return Barbara was just finishing another stanza. I waited for the last "Ah unk!" and opened the curtain. "Here you go. With Mom's permission of course." Mom nodded yes.

After Mom and son left I remarked, "I didn't know you sing. The song was very cute. You've taken lessons in more than pole dancing."

"I told you when we met I was in a choir. Remember?"

"You told me you didn't play an instrument, but I missed that you were a singer. Sorry."

"Yes, it was a church choir. We did a children's concert twice a year. Kids love Little Green Frog."

"Well, something else to endear me to you. This gives me an idea."

———————

After a little over a week we still didn't know much about each other. In any mixture of young men and women, if all you had to go by were brief bios, Barbara and I would likely not be picked as a couple.

> BW, 27, newly-minted nurse, likes to cook and can sing. From Seattle. Only travel outside U.S. has been to Canada. Briefly married to a jerk. Worked part time as pole dancer before and during nursing school. Not Jewish. 5'5", about 130 lbs.
>
> JL, 33, an emergency-medicine doctor originally from Ohio. Never married. Plays guitar, doesn't like to cook. India sojourn before med school. Jewish. 5'11", about 180 lbs.

Of course the relationship was made by the emotional and physical bonding at night, or during the day if either of us worked the night shift. I loved that I could give her multiple climaxes, after which she would get me to the boiling point -- so insane that I would cry out and have to catch myself lest a neighbor complain. But it was more than the sex, it was the mutual appreciation for each other's career, abilities and aspirations. Our brief relationship made me think of and appreciate Mom and Dad.

They must have experienced the same relationship when young, and now they were married forty years. I wanted to be so fortunate. With Barbara I felt there was an excellent chance.

Our first conversation in Melvin's Diner revealed most of what we needed to know. The first night together in bed (before Judy arrived, of course) revealed the rest.

Now it was just fun to learn about our individual likes and dislikes, what interests we might share as the days and years unfolded. The day after her 'Ah unk!' performance I brought home a present.

"For me?" She held the gift-wrapped rectangular-shaped box, shaking to see if it rattled. "Let me guess," she said. "Not jewelry. Too big. Not books. Too light. Not golf clubs. Too short."

"Give up? Open it."

"I know. It has something to do with my singing yesterday. It gave you an idea. I remember, see?"

"You're getting warmer," I offered.

"Let's see, I don't play any instrument, so can't be that. Umm." Curiosity took over and she tore open the wrapping and read the label on the box.

"Kala Concert Ukulele. Josh! I don't play the ukulele."

"I know. Open it."

She removed the uke, along with a thin book of simple songs and instructional chords.

"It's very pretty, she said. I love the wood."

"Koa wood. From Hawaii."

"It's like a little guitar."

"Let me show you." I strummed a few chords, did a quick tuning with an electronic tuner, then handed the uke back to her. "This is the easiest fretted instrument to learn. With your singing background and ability to read music, you can pick it up in no time. I didn't want to ask you first, since I was afraid you'd say no. If you don't like it, no problem. But I think you have talent for this. You'll be amazed how easy it is to learn."

She offered no further objection and began skimming through the booklet. "I haven't looked at music in years," she said. "G Clef. Four-four time. Oh, look. *Clementine* and *Amazing Grace*. Wow, I remember those songs. It's all coming back to me."

She began singling Clementine, without the uke. I picked it up and strummed.

Oh my darling, oh my darling
Oh my darling Clementine
Thou art lost and gone forever,
Dreadful sorry, Clementine

"Wow, you can really sing."

"And you can really play. Leave it out. I'll look at it after supper." She gave me a kiss and went in the kitchen to finish making dinner.

CHAPTER 7

⬩

THE NEXT TWO WEEKS WENT by quickly. Reuniting with Barbara and being rid of Judy made me a happy camper. I also learned that my patient Vicki Ledbetter was taken off the ventilator after two days in the ICU. She had made a full recovery and was discharged home.

In late October we were blessed with gorgeous weather. Barbara and I managed two great hikes in Red Rock Canyon. I should have added 'likes to hike' to her resume.

There were only two blips during this period, neither one what I would call major. One afternoon in the ED I got a text message. "Urgent. Pleeze call. Need help. JB."

I had not changed my cell phone number, had not even thought to do so. If Judy really needed assistance, and I could help without getting re-involved, of course I would. I was still her friend, if not her lover.

I called. "Judy, what's the matter?"

"Oh Josh," she said. "Thanks for calling."

"No problem. What's the matter?" I repeated.

"He's left me. I don't know where to go. What should I do?"

"Who's left you?"

"He has. The guy who lives in your building." Dummy I am, but to that point I just wasn't thinking he was me.

"Josh, ask him to return, won't you? Please. You see him every day. You're the only one who can make him change his mind."

Wow! She was way off the deep end. I was *so* glad she was in California.

"No problem, Judy. I'll see what I can do. Anything else?"

"Let me know as soon as you talk to him."

"OK."

"Promise?"

"I promise. Goodbye Judy."

Right after work I drove to the Verizon store on Maryland Parkway. Now I had not only a new door lock but a new cell phone number. Would I also need a new apartment?

———◆———

The second blip was, in a way, more predictable. My parents called just to say hello, and Barbara answered the phone. I wasn't home, but heard about it later. Barbara felt somewhat embarrassed, but from what I gather handled the call well. She was just a little miffed about having to be the one to tell Mom and Dad about us.

"Was it a secret?" she asked.

"It's only been a week, Barb. I only talk to them about once every two weeks." My logic was unassailable, of course.

"Ten days, just so you know."

"Well, there was no urgency."

"Your Mom seemed puzzled about my last name. Twice she asked, 'Did you say Wilson'? And it wasn't a bad connection. Is Wilson a foreign name in your neighborhood?"

"It'll be fine, Barbara," I said. "I've dated non-Jewish girls before. And don't forget, the last one *was* Jewish."

Later I called home. Mom answered. "We talked to your new girlfriend."

"I know Mom, she told me. Very nice, isn't she?"

"She's not Jewish?"

46

"No, Mom. I broke up with the Jewish one. The one I was dating from LA."

"Oh? That's too bad." It was just the opposite of course, except in the world of Jewish moms.

"You'll like Barbara, I promise."

"So she lives with you?"

"Yes."

"Be careful."

"About what?"

"Just be careful, you know."

"She's not going to get pregnant, don't worry."

"What's her family like?"

Here I was more or less ignorant. Her parents and a sister were ensconced in Seattle. Her parents apparently had come to Vegas only once, for Barbara's graduation from nursing school. Barbara had been back home several times. They were there, she was here, and she seemed happy with the arrangement.

"I haven't met them yet."

"Oh?" I think she thought that was good, maybe indicating Barbara and I weren't too serious. The rest of the conversation was about my sister, niece and nephew, my old neighborhood. Family stuff.

"When are you coming home?" I lived and worked in Las Vegas but my "home" to her was still the place I grew up.

"I don't know. I've been pretty busy. When are you and Dad coming out to Vegas? They're always having medical conventions here."

"Well, if you're not going to come here, I guess maybe we'll have to come to Nevada. I'll talk to your father."

CHAPTER 8

ON NOVEMBER 1ST BARBARA HAD her last pole performance. I had voiced some concern over this side job, as I knew it meant men drooling over her boobs (and other body parts), and because the job was, in my eyes, demeaning. I did not pressure her to quit, but my attitude was the catalyst she needed. I had been home from the hospital only an hour when she walked in.

"I'm done with poles, Honey."

"Thank goodness. Are you OK with your decision?"

"Yes. Enough is enough."

"Good. I'm glad."

"Guess what?" she asked, while changing clothes.

"You're going to give up nursing and make a full career of lap dancing," I said.

"No, silly boy. I'm done, as promised. No poles, no laps. Except yours, of course. No, Irene and Carl made a video of what they call the top ten positions for sex. It's professionally done, and she says it's a big hit on Triple X-Vegas."

"What is Triple X-Vegas?"

"You know, the local porn channel. It's right here in Las Vegas, but syndicated all over the country."

"You watch that stuff?" I asked.

"No, but many of the clients at the club do, as well as probably half the men around this town. Triple X is locally produced, but they compete with half a dozen other cable porn channels. You get them in all the hotel rooms. You're not into this cable porn?"

"I have you," I said, and patted her behind. "Why do I need to watch sex on TV?"

"Good answer. You pass. But now my best friend's on cable, so I am curious. It's pay per view. Do you mind if we watch it tonight?"

Do I mind? My girlfriend is asking *me* to watch porn with *her.* I imagine in 99% of similar situations, it's the guy who wants to watch, and the girlfriend either refuses or goes along reluctantly, or smacks him side of the head and walks out. Of course I said yes, I don't mind at all.

Barbara's friend Irene is just as curvaceous but more, well, extroverted. She seems to have no inhibition in showing off her moves. Here's the shocker, to me at least. She made the video with her *husband.* They've been married a year, no children. Carl Collins is a pit boss at the Argonaut, Vegas's newest luxury hotel extravaganza. Thirty-five hundred rooms, fifteen restaurants, and a casino the size of three football fields.

Before marrying Irene he did some videos for Triple X-Vegas. This new video was his idea, apparently fully endorsed by his wife. When Carl suggested they share their bedtime escapades with anyone willing to pay a few bucks to watch, she didn't hesitate. Barbara quoted me Irene's justification: "Why not make some money off what we do almost every night?"

"How much?" I asked.

"Don't know, but I imagine it could be substantial," said Barbara. "The channel itself is $20/month to subscribers, and each pay per view is $9.99. Next time I see her I'll ask if they're planning to retire."

"Imagine that," I chimed in, "being able to retire because of a video made screwing your wife. Everyone should be making these videos. It's fun, it's legal and you can retire! Whoopee."

"It makes money because everyone is *not* making them," she said. "Do you want to show your thing to the world? I don't. There has to be some pride."

"Oh, darn," I said, "you mean I have to keep practicing medicine?" She laughed.

Barbara found the cable channel and after pressing half a dozen buttons, and entering my credit card number, we watched "Top 10 Positions: Let Sasha and Boris show you how." Irene and Carl used aliases but the video showed their real bodies.

"How did they do this with all those cameramen around?" There were two camera angles, so I assumed there was more than one. This was not an amateur production.

"Just two, she told me. Irene says it's done in a soundproof room at the studio, where they film a lot of porn. All the equipment is there already. The two camera guys are dressed in black, and Irene said you don't even notice them after a while. The biggest problem is the lighting; it blunts some of the romance."

"She told you all this? You two must have had quite a conversation."

"She likes to talk. I like to listen. It's always been that way."

"Are you suggesting something about our relationship?"

"Aren't I a good listener?"

We had somehow digressed. "What else did she say?"

"She said it took them four nights of shooting to make the thing. There's only so many times you can have sex in two hours. She has a saying. 'Once is fun, two is enough, three is work and four is painful'. I think they stopped after two or three times."

I won't enumerate the positions in the video, but you can imagine. There was fore-play, intra-play, after-play. There was, thankfully, no voice over or music, but the video did employ short textual labels, e.g., REVERSE STRADDLE POSITION. This was not simulated sex and you could hear the moans, squeaks and squeals of lovemaking. The quality was there, but I was otherwise unimpressed. "Who's going to buy this shit?" I asked. The question just popped into my head.

"You are, Honey, we are. We just did."

"If guys have to watch this to learn how to fuck, they're beyond help," I said. Actually, some of the positions were acrobatic, and I could not do them without self-inflicted bodily harm. I was glad Barbara didn't insist on trying out all ten in this video.

"So it doesn't turn you on?" she asked, while her right hand unzipped my pants.

"No, but you turn me on."

"Do you think we could make a video?" she asked, her hand now firmly around its target and massaging gently.

"Of what, you dancing about my pole?"

"How about your patient's elimination contest?"

"Why would anyone want to watch that?"

"Same answer, Honey. You did. We did. The place was packed."

"If it's such a good idea, how come it's not already on Triple X?" I asked.

"Don't think they know about it," she said. "Probably the best kept secret in Vegas. Is there any other activity so under the radar?"

By this time I was almost ready to explode, and rolled over to finish what she started. I joked, "Position seven."

She joked back. "Roger, position seven." I don't remember what position seven was, but it didn't matter. What did matter was that, while making love, I could not get out of my mind her comment, "under the radar." *Why were contests at Joe's Plumbing Supplies so under the radar? The Biggest Loser was a hit TV show, based on dieting. Would a wider audience be interested in weight loss after a single bathroom break?* And at the same time, I had a parallel thought – *Why do I care?*

———◆———

Nothing more came of this thought until three nights later, when we had dinner with Carl and Irene. We'd been out with them once before, at the Argonaut. Since he worked there, the dinner had been comp'd. I did leave a nice tip though. On this second outing, we went to a restaurant at Ariel, and split the check.

I did not particularly like Carl. He started out in Vegas as a blackjack dealer, moved his way up to pit boss and now supervised a quadrant of blackjack tables at the Argonaut. Pit bosses and a gazillion video cameras are the prime methods of preventing cheating – by dealers and patrons.

He seemed too smooth to me. His hair, speech, clothes – all polished. I had my own theory on this. At work he was always on camera, and therefore always on guard. He never knew when the casino bosses might be looking at him through endless loops of the same video. And perhaps, even away from the pit, they were checking him out to see if he could move up to floor manager. My theory sounded good, but more likely Carl *became* an effective pit boss because he was Mr. Smoothie -- long before he ever entered a casino.

Irene loved him, though, which was the all-important thing. And Barbara and Irene were best friends. The husband of my live-in girl-friend's best friend is my friend, so Carl and I actually got along well on our double dates. But without the female connection, nada.

"We enjoyed your video," Barbara said.

Back where I grew up, this comment would elicit utter embarrassment. *You saw a video of me and hubby fucking? Oh, I'm so embarrassed.*

Not here, not Irene and Carl. They were pleased. "Yes," said Irene, "it's actually doing quite well. We've made some money already." I was not gauche enough to ask how much.

"I was telling Josh about Triple X," Barbara said. "He never heard of it."

"Local porn cable," replied Carl. "Low budget but they do a good job. You two should check it out. You look like the kind of studs they want on Triple X."

"I don't think so," said Barbara. "Actually, we saw an act the other night that might find a home on Triple X."

"Oh?" said Carl.

"Tell him, honey."

This is how it started. Just conversation. The smoothie and the doctor. I summarized the contest night, evincing a hint of disgust which I thought would be shared by all. I didn't want Carl and Irene to think *I* go for this entertainment.

"How many people did you say were there?"

"We estimated about seventy-five," said Barbara.

"And betting?"

"You bet," she said. We all laughed.

"Hmmm," said Carl. "What do you think, Irene?"

"Sounds disgusting to me," she said.

"Do you guys know about the pissing contests?"

"You mean literally pissing?" I asked, "Or just when people get into a verbal shouting match."

"The literal kind," said Carl.

"Seems to ring a bell of some sort. I think one of the fraternities at college had one."

"Yeah, it's definitely a sophomore thing," said Carl. "But for a while they were having formal pissing contests in Vegas, in people's backyards, with organized betting. The longest distance won."

"And?"

"Well, it's the same thing. People bet on how far you can piss, how much stuff you can excrete. They'll bet on anything."

"Barbara and I likened it to cockfighting. Anything to get your juices up, even better if the authorities frown on it."

"No, my point," Carl said, now getting pedantic on us, "is that it's not much different than roulette or blackjack or slot machines. There's some metric: a distance, a weight, a group of numbers, a series of cards. You think you have the answer, or can find the winner, and you bet. Down deep you know the odds are against you, but it doesn't seem to matter. It's fun. It interests people. Always has and always will."

"So you're interested?" I asked.

"Personally, no, I don't give a crap," Carl said, "but Gabe Stein might be."

CHAPTER 9

———

LAS VEGAS IS NOT LIKE any other city in America. On one level it's a typical town, whose main industries happen to be gambling and tourism. It has the same urban problems as any large metropolis (crime, traffic, congestion, pollution, homelessness), and offers the same services vital for any city to function (fire, police, medical, trash pickup).

On another level Vegas is atypical because it tolerates – indeed, fosters – activities which in any other town would be eschewed or condemned. Vegas is the most libertarian town in America; it allows people like Jack Strawn, Barbara Wilson, and Gabe Stein, proprietor of Triple X Las Vegas, to come and do their own thing, and no one cares. It's not just "What happens here stays here." It's more like "What happens here is your own damn business." That I might be the exception to this rule never, ever dawned on me.

Carl and I drove together to meet Gabe. Along the way he warned me: "He's from New York and sometimes hard to understand."

I'll say. Gabe's "you" became "youse," "talk" changed to "tawk" and "thirty" sound "toidy." I can't write the way he talked, so in print it will sound normal.

I estimated Gabe to be in his mid-50s. He was thin, sported long uncombed hair and a faint goatee. He wore a Hawaiian-style shirt open at the collar, showing a little bit of upper chest hair. He also sported one of those five pound gold bracelets on his left wrist. Good thing he was right-handed. As soon as we entered the office he came from behind a large desk to shake our hands and said "take a seat," accented in a way to suggest we should pick up a chair and carry it home.

"Tell me your idea," Gabe said.

Somehow Barbara's idea had become my idea and now Mr. Stein wanted to know about it. Carl had set up the meeting and I agreed to go out of curiosity, more to learn about Triple X than any real desire to promote instant Biggest Loser contests. All things Vegas interested me, and this was just another opportunity to learn more about my new hometown. Carl had already explained to Gabe what I told him at the restaurant.

"Quite frankly, Mr. Stein," I said, "we're not sure if there is anything here to interest your demographic."

"What is my demographic?"

I looked at Carl for guidance.

"Joshua means, men who watch sex."

"Well, let me be the judge of that," Stein replied. "You'd be amazed who watches what."

"My girlfriend and I just happened to be invited to an elimination contest at a local strip mall," I said. "They held it at Joe's Plumbing Supplies, which apparently, for some reason, is equipped with about ten bathrooms, one for each contestant. They had three rounds, and cleaned 'em between contests. Guys with mops stood by. There was all sorts of betting and a lot of audience interest. They seemed to be having a good time, albeit over a bathroom activity. There's no sex involved."

"We can do without the sex. Tell me more."

I told him about Jack Strawn, but made no mention about his being a one-time patient. I said he was an acquaintance.

"Your acquaintance, is he black or white?"

"White. Does it matter?"

"Depends. We show plenty of beautiful black women and handsome black men. And we show black on white, white on black, doesn't matter. They all look good. But your act is different. If these guys are all black and the act bombs, I could be accused of exploitation. Don't need that aggravation. How many spectators did you say were there?"

"About seventy-five. It was standing room only. They have these contests about once or twice a week, I gather."

"Always at Joe's Plumbing?"

"Apparently so. The guy's got three stores in the metro area, but all the contests are in the central store on South Decatur."

"Makes sense," said Gabe. "The guy sells toilets. I've heard of this before. Sort of underground. Not publicized."

"That's right."

"There might be a place on my network for such an act. But for women contestants."

"Women?"

"Yes. No one's going to be that much interested in fat men losing weight in the bathroom. You're describing The Biggest Losers. Ever see the show?"

"Yes," I said. "Everyone makes the comparison."

"Well, they have women and men. But in my business, it's really women, then men. Do you get the distinction?"

I assumed his demographic was mostly men, but did not answer.

"Anyway, he continued, get me women, in bikinis or less, and the ratings will shoot up. Then I can also have men, men vs. women. I like the idea."

"Interesting you bring that up, Mr. Stein."

"Josh, Josh, call me Gabe. You're a *landsman.* Let's be informal."

"OK, Gabe. The night we went to see the contest, I learned they had tried it before with women, and it didn't work out. It is a male thing as far as contestants go."

"Probably because it's a live performance," said Stein. "Everyone's packed into one area, as you describe it. Men probably want to go feel up the girls, or oogle their boobs. Not a good scene. I can see where it would get out of hand." He paused for a thought. "But it might work on live remote video. Or better yet, on a stage where the audience is more separated. That is, of course, if the women are willing."

"Do you have enough bathrooms?" I asked. "Joe's has lot of bathrooms. The night we went they handled fifteen contestants, each with his own toilet, apparently. Do you have enough for a live performance?"

"*Not* a problem," Gabe shot back. "Just need three contestants at a time. Can handle it easily. We can clean bathrooms just as quickly as Joe with his mop guys. What else?"

"Why don't you explain the financials to the doctor?" asked Carl.

"Good idea. We have 110,000 national subscribers. They are pretty hard core. We show sex of course, everything from anal to blow jobs. You can stream it on your computer or watch it on television. Late at night we have homosexuality, but not during prime time. Not good for the kids." He laughed.

"We have done pissing contests. We have done contests based on time to ejaculation from both blow jobs and masturbation. We have real world videos of people fucking while sky diving, scuba diving, water skiing. Do you know how hard it is to screw while water skiing?"

"Can't imagine," I said.

"People watch this shit, what can I say? Do you know the difference between what's porn and what's not porn?" Gabe directed the question to me. I vaguely remembered something about a Supreme Court you-know-it-when-you-see-it decision, but didn't think that was what he was looking for.

"No."

"Porn is a public showing of what people do in private."

I did not respond, but didn't need to. Gabe was on some kind of roll.

"Tell me," he said. "How come you can watch on TV, or in the movies, people being killed, tortured, maimed, chopped up, sliced and diced, but you can't watch the normal human sex act? Why is sex pornography, but murder and mayhem are not? I mean, it's great for my business, since it drives the content underground and increases the fee structure. I'd be dead if CBS and NBC showed fucking every night. But I never figured out how we came to glorify blood and guts in mainstream media, but can't show a man and woman screwing."

"You have a good point, Mr. Stein," I said. He really did, but being a mainstream kind of guy myself, I had no desire to buck common cultural norms. And besides, I personally never watched porn, preferring the real thing to what I could see on a screen.

"Anyway, where was I?" asked Gabe. "Oh, yeah. Get me women who will appear in bikinis and I think there's a market. We can add the men later. Men versus women. But first start with the women. Bosomy women. And on the younger side, not over forty. I don't care if they're fat. Fat is attractive too, to some men."

Of course I had no idea what sort of women once tried out as contestants. I assumed they were not grandmothers.

"You'll get a percentage as agent," Gabe continued. "As for a live show, live shows are expensive. We have a small auditorium, but a live show requires a host, two cameramen, assistants to arrange the acts, bouncers to keep the audience in check. We've done audience shows before, but it's way more labor intensive than pre-shot or even live streamed video. I could consider a live show if one or both of you put up investor money. Then we'd split the profits, depending on how much you put up."

Carl waved off. "No thanks, Gabe. I've got my hands full with the casino. Don't want to call any attention to the Gaming Commission."

"You mean this isn't legal?" I asked.

"One hundred percent legal, Josh. You think I'd be running this business with 110 thousand subscribers if it wasn't legal? No, Carl means he can't invest in any operation related to betting, since he works for a casino."

"The show has betting?"

"Whenever we have contests, like the pissing match I told you about, an affiliate of ours conducts on-line betting. We as cable producer take a percentage. Since it's all local, it's all legal. But it would be a conflict for Carl."

"So if we set up women in a defecation contest, there would be sideline betting?"

"Yes, of course. Not the live audience members, since the process would be too unwieldy on a live cable show. But from the internet crowd, definitely. If a guy is jerking off in front of his computer, he can also place a bet at the same time. Wonderful, this technology, isn't it?"

"But the video would be history by the time it's shown. Surely people will already know the outcome and influence the betting."

"Of course, of course, Josh. The betting could only work in a live show. A truly, 100% live show. Then, it could rake in a lot of money."

"And the money would be split fifty-fifty?"

"For that particular show, yes, depending on how much you, as investor, put up."

"How much are you talking about?"

"For a live show?"

"Yes." Despite all my questions, I still felt, indeed was certain, that I was *merely curious*. I was in a foreign culture, talking business with a native about whom I knew almost nothing. In truth, I was getting in way over my head, but could not stop. Barbara didn't stop me from going to this meeting. Carl didn't stop me. My parents were nowhere around to hold my hand. I was just asking questions, which Stein seemed more than happy to answer. He scribbled some numbers on a piece of paper.

"If we produce an hour-long show, say once a week, with the usual potpourri of sex, and add contests with your ladies, let's see. I could put together a production crew, announcer, cameramen. We would plan for about six shows altogether, to see if it catches on. We already have the space for an audience of about 200. Not large, but enough to give the show some sparkle, generate interest. Sort of like Jerry Springer, but far raunchier, depending on your point of view. We could out do Springer! A hundred thou could get us started."

"Total?"

"No, no. 100K would be your investment. It would guarantee six shows. You would get half the profits and any residuals afterwards, for reruns. Of course the betting would only be during the live shows."

"I am a doctor, not a businessman, so I have no feel for this type of deal." *What an understatement.* "It is intriguing, though."

"Yeah, think about it. But in the meantime, find me some women willing to participate. I'll take the guys too, but only after the women do at least one or two shows. I envision a man vs. woman Biggest Loser contest. No dieting needed. This is great. I *like* the idea. You will get ten percent as agent."

"What about Carl?" I asked. "He set up this meeting."

"He works for a casino. Can't get involved in any outside betting activity. Carl and I have other arrangements, so he's covered."

I didn't ask what they were. "I understand, but please explain. Ten percent of what?"

"As agent, ten percent of what I pay the people you find for me, if they sign on."

"And what do you pay?"

"Union wages. Generally, $500 a show."

"So if my acquaintance appears once a week on your show for six weeks, he will receive 3,000 dollars?"

"Right, and you would get 300. It's simple."

"But if I invest in the show, there's royalties?"

"That's a whole different ball of cotton fiber," he said. "Now we're talking investment. You then become a co-producer, share all the royalties. It's a longer contract."

"I'll talk to my acquaintance. This has certainly been interesting, Mr. Stein. Vegas has more layers than I ever imagined. Pole dancing, defecation contests, porn channels."

"We don't do pole dancing. Doesn't work on video," said Stein. "And *please*, call me Gabe. It will be a pleasure working with you. And you too, of course, Carl. And say hello to that lovely wife of yours."

Carl nodded. It was time to go.

CHAPTER 10

—◆—

SIX MONTHS BEFORE MY RESIDENCY ended I flew out to Vegas to interview for the Memorial ED job. My first and most important interview was with Dr. John Billington, president of the hospital. An orthopedic surgeon by training, he had had obtained an MBA in his forties and gone into hospital administration, becoming Memorial's Chief Executive Officer a decade earlier. In ten years he had changed Memorial from a 350-bed community hospital to a 600-bed major medical center, and was somewhat revered in the annals of hospital CEO's. This accomplishment was greatly abetted by Vegas' growth in population and tourism, and the massive amount of money available for hospital construction. Almost every wing was named for a casino mogul. Doctors make a good living, but it's small potatoes compared to these guys; when they give $20 million for a new surgical suite, it's like me giving $200 to United Way. It affects our bottom line about the same.

Dr. Billington was a handsome guy, regal looking you might say, tall with a head of Trump-like hair. On the day I met him he wore a suit, a rarity, it seemed, among the power elite of Vegas. Before the interview he had read my CV, knew I was from Ohio and had taken two years off between college and medical school.

"Why the hiatus?" he asked.

I told him the story, and was happy to learn he, too, had spent some time in India on a medical lecture circuit. Different experiences, to be sure. I felt certain he had never studied in an ashram or toured the country by bus, as I had. Still, we had been to some of the same cities, seen the same sites. The interview was a snap from then on.

"So why do you want to come to Las Vegas?" he asked.

"Well, first, I am impressed with your hospital, think the ED provides a great professional opportunity." Of course there were hundreds like it throughout the country, but when you praise the CEO's accomplishment he's not going to be critical. "And I am looking for a change of scenery."

"Well, you're not alone. Do you know half the population here is from somewhere else? I'm from Denver myself. Did you get our pay package?"

The job offered $250,000 a year, with a two year contract, and included health insurance and pension plan. This was of course more money than I ever imagined making. "Yes," I said, "seems very reasonable." I had heard through the grapevine that Dr. Billington made over one million a year. Administration always seems to pay better than patient care.

"Other doctors in your family?" he asked.

"Well, my father, he's an orthopedic surgeon in Cleveland."

"He is? What's his name?" I told him.

"Gerald Luvkin is your father?"

Turns out my dad had published some medical articles on a new hip joint, about ten years ago. He was sort of well-known among academic orthopedists for this reason, and before becoming CEO, Dr. Billington was in that group. For the next five minutes we played orthopedic-surgeon geography, who knew whom, etc. By the end of the interview we were best buddies and I knew I had the job. I still had two more interviews to go, with the chairman of the department of surgery and an ED physician, but they were perfunctory.

Two weeks after returning home I got a contract from the hospital. A little over three years later I had my first date with Barbara.

I never regretted taking the Memorial Hospital job. Besides the good pay, the hospital offers great patient care and excellent camaraderie among the staff. Memorial has a powerhouse of specialists who often come to our aid in the ED. The specialists typically arrive with a team, like swat teams. A heart problem in the ED? Call the cardiology swat team. At least the cardiology fellow and resident will come pronto. Sometimes the head physician will also show up. In this way I got to know Dr. Clarence Meringhaus, Chief of the Pulmonary Division, who also happens to head the hospital's Ethics Department. I liked and trusted Clarence, which is why I called him the day after my visit with Gabe Stein.

"Clarence, I have an ethics question for you. Do you have a minute?"

"Sure. Shoot."

"I saw a patient in the ED last month, who operates a business. He has a certain skill that people bet on. It's all probably legal, I don't know, but that's beside the point. I've since learned that a friend of mine wants to hire him for this skill, to produce a show of sorts, and wants me to arrange a meeting. If my friend hires him I will get a percentage of what my ex-patient receives, as an agent's fee. Am I permitted to contact my ex-patient and inform him of this opportunity?"

A straight forward question, it seemed to me, but not with an obvious answer. Physicians have to be careful about violating any HIPPA laws, or running afoul of a hospital's ethics guidelines. My generation of physicians is hyperaware.

"He is not your patient on an on-going basis?

"Nope, just saw him the one time for an acute arthritic condition. We don't have any ongoing doctor-patient relationship. He has his own medical doctor."

"Did you know him before the encounter?"

"No, never saw him before."

"Do you plan to divulge the money you will make if he signs with your friend?"

"Of course. I have nothing to hide."

"But your ex-patient, he would potentially make money off this arrangement?"

"I hope so. I should add, he already uses his skill to make extra money after his regular day job, so he's somewhat of an entrepreneur. My own sense is he would jump at this opportunity if he knew about it. So one could argue it might be unethical *not* to inform him. However, that's not my question. Is it ethical to contact him? I just want your opinion. And I know what you might be thinking, so let me make it clear his activity is not male prostitution or anything to do with sex. And I'm certain the job he would be hired for is legal."

There was a pause, and I could hear some throat clearing. I trusted Clarence not to hem and haw and waste my time on philosophical musings. He was known for incisive thinking. Also, I was not asking for a legal opinion.

"Josh, the short answer is yes, it's ethical to contact him and explain the opportunity. I would feel much less comfortable if you had an ongoing relationship with him, but as an ED doc I know you don't. So that's the short answer."

"And the long answer?"

"The long answer is, if it doesn't work out, are you putting yourself in jeopardy for a bad reputation? The long answer is, why do you want to get involved in anything even peripherally related to gambling? The long answer is, do you know what you're doing?"

All good questions, for which I didn't have any good answers.

CHAPTER 11

—————

Here is a generalization I believe to be true. When doctors go outside their profession to make money, for all their smarts they are at a big disadvantage. Consider just these money-seeking activities tried by colleagues I know.

* Owning, and helping to manage, a restaurant
* Writing a novel
* Writing a screenplay
* Real estate investment in an apartment building
* Running an e-Bay business
* Collecting and trading sports memorabilia
* Buying and rehabilitating antique cars

There are common themes in these endeavors. They all began after the physicians entered medical practice, when they had accumulated disposable income. All the physicians hoped to make a profit. All the endeavors are time consuming. And all are dominated by professionals who spend way more time on them then the physician can.

So why do doctors strive for these side careers? For some, a hobby turns into a business and they can't let go (car restoration comes to mind). Others see the activity as an escape from their medical career, perhaps leading to early retirement.

Of course, you don't see writers, real estate investors or car collectors entering the medical field, because medicine is a rigorous profession. It requires special training and certification. But while you don't need certification to write a novel, that doesn't mean it's easy. Ditto everything else on the list. Yet some doctors feel they can enter other professions through the back door, as it were, and succeed. The truth is, far more often than not, they fail.

Why did I think I would be different?

I called Jack Strawn. He was surprised to hear from me.

"I was your doctor at Memorial, when you came in with the gout."

"Sure, I remember you? Did you get to my contest? I won my section."

"Yes, I did. So how is your gout?"

"Much better, much better Doc. Is that why you're calling?"

"Well, it's one reason. But actually there's another reason. I met someone who is interested in your contests, and I want to discuss it with you. It's kind of complicated. Could we meet for lunch?"

"You buying?"

"Of course. How about Melvin's Diner?"

"Great food, great food."

We arranged to meet the next day. I hoped I could afford his lunch.

One of the other nice things about Melvin's -- apart from the quiet ambience -- is the menu. It's humungous, but well-categorized. Every time I go there I'm reminded of Arlo Guthrie's song *Alice's Restaurant*, which isn't about a restaurant or food but does contain a refrain about being able to get anything you want at "Alice's Restaurant." I've thought about writing a folk song, *Melvin's Restaurant.* In my spare time.

"So, what's up Doc?"

"I'll tell you in a minute. Let's order first."

He stared at the menu for just a second, then said, "Know what I want."

I called the waitress over. Normally, given the size of the menu, they give you five-ten minutes to figure things out. We were ready in less than a minute.

She came over and Jack said, "I'll have the five-egg omelet, with bacon and cheddar, order of rye toast, order of hash browns, and a side of blueberry pancakes. And orange juice and coffee."

"Are you ordering for both of you?"

"Uh, no," I said. "That's just for him."

She smiled.

"I'll have the two-egg omelet, with Swiss, and an order of wheat toast. No fries. And also orange juice and coffee." She left with the orders.

"They have great omelets here," said Jack. "So, what's up?"

I went right into the whole history: my trip to his contest (did not mention Barbara, though), my conversation with spectators, my connection with Gabe Stein, and Stein's interest in the contests. Strawn listened as attentively as any struggling performer might, who has a chance to enter the big top.

"Sounds very interesting," he said.

"There's only one catch," I said.

"Which is?"

"This guy Stein, who runs the cable channel. He wants women."

"There's plenty of women in Vegas. Is he married?"

"No, no, I'm not explaining myself. He wants women contestants. For the elimination contests. He wants women first, then will consider men, possibly even a men vs. women contest."

"We tried women before. Doesn't work. Men in the audience start doing catcalls. They yell for them to take off the bikini tops. Women get intimidated. Then the gals in the audience get pissed and start fighting with their boyfriends or whatever. It doesn't work."

"He thinks it might."

"How so?"

"Either through live video, or a studio arrangement with a better separation of contestants and audience. He has ideas."

"Then, where do I come in?"

"Can you find women contestants, willing to go on what's essentially a porn channel?"

"They paying?"

"Of course"

"How much?"

"He says $500 a show. There will be betting, but I don't think the contestants share in the pot. Actually, I'm not sure, now that I think about it. Certainly this is something probably negotiable."

"Who does the negotiating?"

"I guess we do."

"We? You mean me and you are partners?"

Up to this point I had no business plan, no contract, and no experience in anything we talked about. I was ad-libbing. But it made sense that the contestants should get something from the pot. It also made sense that Strawn and I work together in negotiations. He should be on my side, rather than worry about any adversarial relationship. All these things made sense. Still, there is no way around the fact I was winging it, as they say.

"Well, not exactly partners, but work together, sort of, to see if we can get this idea moving along."

"I am still not sure what you want me to do, doc." He was getting a little annoyed over my bumbling. I had to be more assertive.

"OK. Let me try to focus. Find willing women contestants. Not grandmothers, either. They can be heavy – hell, they should be heavy – but need to be television pretty. Tell them they'll each get $500 a show, possibly more if it works out, but no promises. When you get a list, you and I, together, will go to Triple X and negotiate with Mr. Stein. We'll see what he's willing to offer. I can't make any promises. I've only met the man once. We'll split whatever fee I get as the agent here. Gabe's promised me ten percent, but if we cut a good deal with him, there could be some money. Stein is also mighty interested in a men-versus-women contest, which could happen pretty quick if the gals are successful."

Now I had his attention. I sweated a little, autonomic juice anyone with a conscience would feel when making such a flimsy proposal. Consider the odds. Strawn had to find bosomy, attractive women willing to show their blubber on TV and be weighed before and after a trip to the bathroom. The viewers – in whatever medium they chose -- had to like the contest and be induced to bet. Finally, Gabe Stein had to produce the show in a manner to generate good word-of-mouth and make money. All the while, I had to be behind the scenes, as I continued my day (and night) job in the ED.

The food came and I watched Jack eat. He was a sight to behold. I was not yet halfway through my own omelet when he was ready to order dessert.

CHAPTER 12

———◆———

I PICKED UP JACK AND drove him to the meeting with Gabe Stein. On the way he told me he was skeptical of "this porn shit," and I don't think he intended any pun when he said it. He didn't expect to make any real money, and agreed to the meeting as much out of curiosity (like me!) as any real desire to do contests. However, he also had some valuable information: the names and contact information of three buxom women willing to appear on Stein's porn channel.

After introductions Stein asked us to please sit down, but the office chair was too small for Jack.

"This chair ain't gonna work, Mr. Stein," he said.

Fortunately there was a couch across the room, which fit him well. Stein even moved over to us and sat in a chair, so we could talk comfortably.

Jack had gone to junior college for one year, then did a series of odd jobs before landing as a building super in Summerlin. He was what you would call street smart, and did not intimidate easily. Not that Stein tried intimidation; he did not. But whereas I was out of my element in the first two meetings with Stein, Jack was in his comfort zone.

"What are you planning, Mr. Stein? I've got the women, no problem, tell me what you have in mind."

I was more or less peripheral to the conversation. Jack and Gabe talked about a Biggest Loser contest to mimic the one on family TV, but based on elimination and not dieting. They talked about whether the women might appear without a bikini top. Jack was non-committal.

They talked about pitting men against women and running superman and superwoman contests for the top weight loser of all time. Whenever Stein raised a question about this or that possibility, Jack had the same answer: "Possible, could work."

There was some synergy between the two men. But so far, no discussion of money had come up. Then it did.

"So how much are you proposing to pay?"

"Union wages, $500 per woman per appearance."

"And a percentage of the betting?"

"No, I'm afraid that's not possible. We don't give our actors a percentage of the betting proceeds. Don't go there; it's off the table." Strawn did not argue this point, but then said,

"In that case, since there will be betting, my women will take $1000 per show."

"Come again?" said Stein.

"Contestants get a percentage of the pot now, at our contests. So if they're going to be on cable, and the union rate is $500, they need to be compensated for not splitting the pot."

"But as I understand it," said Stein, "their current percentage is zero, since women are kept from even doing your gig."

"Correct. And they're happy to keep not doing it. They're not going to expose themselves for 500 smackers, while you're making money off 'em with betting. Course, you could find your own women, it's a free country, but I think I know more about this sport than most people. And these women trust me."

Strawn was impressive, in effect telling Stein to put up or shut up.

"Well, I am interested in your women contestants, I admit. But the show could bomb. I'll agree to $1000 per contest, only on a per contest basis. No long term contract."

"That's cool. Only they are to be paid at the conclusion of each contest, no 'check's in the mail' BS."

"Mr. Strawn, I run a legitimate operation," Stein said, a little too insouciantly, I thought.

"I trust that, but I don't want to be bothered by them hounding me where's the money. So this helps me too."

"Fair enough. $1000 per woman contestant at the conclusion of each contest."

"Now what about the men?" asked Strawn.

There ensued a discussion about men vs. women. Jack assured Gabe there were plenty of men available and willing to participate, including himself, and they would demand equal wages. He and Gabe agreed that if the women were successful, Stein might try men vs. women later in the series.

So far, the plan was only for live streaming video. Nothing was decided about a live audience or a variety show. Before leaving, Gabe asked me to call him the next day, to discuss that very issue.

I drove Jack back to his home in North Vegas.

"That was pretty impressive," I said, "the way you handled Gabe."

"Wasn't anything. All these porn guys are money grubbers." I was hoping he wouldn't make a Jewish comment. He didn't. "He'll make money off this shit, so an extra 500 bucks is nothing to him."

"I've been meaning to ask you something," I said. "How'd this get started at Joe's Plumbing?"

"That's a story, he said."

He told it almost non-stop, which I will summarize, omitting Jack's many four-letter words. A couple of years ago, one of Joe's regular customers, a plumbing contractor, weighed himself on a bathroom scale at the store. He then went to use the john, and afterwards weighed himself again. When Joe came over, the guy, who was at least a 300-pounder, remarked to Joe he had lost eight pounds "just in your store." Joe challenged him, said that wasn't possible. So the guy returned the next day, and did it again, this time under Joe's close observation of the before and after weights. Overnight the man had consumed half a dozen hotdogs and fries, plus a whole chocolate cream pie, just to make sure he had something to dump at Joe's.

Joe asked a fat friend if he could beat this customer's weight loss, and the friend couldn't. Over a few weeks, he challenged a few other hefty people to try. One guy beat it at 8.5 lbs. Joe then asked the contractor customer if *he* could beat 8.5 lbs. Next thing you know, they have a contest, held after store hours. Joe sensed there was betting potential, and began inviting others to compete. He had at the time two bathrooms in the store. When he had three guys, no one wanted to use a bathroom previously used by another contestant. What's a plumbing supply store owner to do?

Joe began adding bathrooms in his mid-town store, which was a legitimate business expense. In each he installed a different manufacturer's toilet and sink, with a spec sheet on the door listing the brand inside. Now, during the day Joe could show his customers actual working models of ten different toilets and sinks: two models each of Kohler, American Standard, Toto, Bristan, and Regent. At night, the rooms served the contestants. It was a win-win for Joe Calabane, who now had both a deductible business expense and income from the betting.

Jack told the story with some awe. "Smart businessman, this guy Joe."

"Do you think he pays taxes on what he takes in from these contests?" I asked.

Jack laughed. "Do you think I pay taxes? In case you didn't notice, this isn't a credit card business. Cash only."

I felt a little uneasy about his bravado.

CHAPTER 13

———

I DIDN'T HAVE TO CALL Gabe. He called me first.

"Josh, great meeting your friend yesterday," he said over the phone. "I want to talk to you about the variety show. I think this contest with the women has real potential, and want to make it part of the studio show we discussed."

"That's a good idea," I said.

"I want you to be an investor."

"This is the show where I would put up $100,000?"

"Yes, just what we discussed. Can you come to the studio in the next day or so and let's talk about it?"

I could not say no. Like Curious George the monkey, I let my curiosity lead me down paths best left untraveled. We met the next day and he regaled me with the possibility of porn riches.

"With betting on the ladies, and other side bets we do," I see the possibility of 100K profit on each show. With your fifty percent stake, over six shows you could make 300,000. Quadruple your investment in a little over a month.

Per the doctor stereotype, I may be financially unsophisticated but I am not stupid.

"If there is so much potential profit, why do you want an investor at all? I imagine coming up with another 100K on your own isn't difficult."

"Josh, Josh," he said. "It's an investment. All investments are risky. You could make 300,000 profit or lose the entire 100K. Nothing is guaranteed.

Furthermore, did you ever try to borrow money from a bank for a porn show? Good luck. Yeah, I could get the money from some friends down-town who specialize in cement, but I don't want to go there. If you lose 100 thou, I don't have to worry about a one way trip to the desert."

I got his meaning. I represented a no-threat investor. The guys downtown whose names end in vowels would not be. And banks were out of the question. So his pitch did make sense, which for some reason felt reassuring.

Later I discussed Gabe's proposition with Barbara and Carl. Barbara was non-committal, said it was my money but was surprised I'd saved so much in three years.

I had actually saved a little over this amount because I spent very little: apartment rent, food, some money on musical instruments and entertainment, and very little on clothes. I drove my father's Buick se-dan that he gave me during residency. This "old man's car" was quite serviceable in Vegas. Didn't have to worry about nicks and dents in-curred in the parking lot, and insurance on the vehicle was certainly cheaper than if I had a new BMW or Lexus, which most doctors seemed to drive. And Nevada has no state income taxes. All in all, a single guy with a high income can save a lot in Vegas, and I did. Now, I was willing to risk the fruits of my prudence.

"That's it," I said. "If I lose it I start over, but I've got a lot of years left."

"Well, if you think it's possible to make that much profit, go for it," she said. "Goodness knows, doctors have invested in a lot worse."

"They have?" I asked. "Like what?" She couldn't think of anything worse.

Carl was more enthusiastic, but wary about the contract. "If you get a contract, you'll need a lawyer. Don't sign anything without showing it to my attorney. He's done business with Triple X before and has helped me. It's all business, remember. You need a good contract lawyer." At that point I was glad I knew Mr. Smoothie, who seemed to have the an-swers about all things Vegas.

————

In the midst of this new wrinkle in my life, a wonderful thing happened. Barbara began playing the ukulele. Just as I had promised, the chords came easy. Her singing ability gave tremendous advantage, as what's a good song without the singing? With just five chords under her belt she was a knockout performer. In my apartment, that is. Now she had to become comfortable jamming with others.

Vegas is not a folk music town. There are a few venues where you can hear Irish-type folk, but none that caters to what is now called American Roots music. There is one place, however, perfect for me – when I could get there.

Gilligan's Coffee and Bistro is owned and operated by a guitar player who jammed in college, like me. Every Thursday night John Gilligan opened up his back room for people to meet and jam to their hearts' content, or at least for a couple of hours. The room is big enough for about ten musicians and fifty patrons. There was no charge. You could order food before the performance or just come to listen.

Publicity was all word of mouth, plus a notice on his restaurant's internet page. The few times I went, there were several guitars, a mandolin, two banjos and one banjolele. Once a guy brought a tenor ukulele to play. We belted out songs we knew, then took audience suggestions.

The only problem from my perspective was availability on Thursdays at 9 pm. I was usually either working or post-call. As result, I made it to Gilligan's at most once every month or two. I wanted to take Barbara to the next session, so she had to be off work as well. Finally a Thursday came when we could both go, the week before Thanksgiving.

"Bring your ukulele."

"I hardly know the thing," she said.

"You're too modest. You know enough to participate. I've heard you. You'll like it. Sit in the audience, just listen. If you know the song, sing it. This is really, really low key," I said. The tickets are cheap.

"Yes, you told me. When I play they'll ask for a refund." What a sense of humor my Barbara has!

———◆———

Gilligan's is popular with the locals, an alternative to Starbucks and Panera. Located in the Charleston Heights area, the main dining room is spacious and comfortable, with superb coffee and sandwiches. The bistro uses a large back room for private parties several times a month.

I was the most irregular of the regulars for the Thursday night jams, and the only physician in the group.

"Welcome back, Doc. Where you been?"

"Working. Playing all the great rooms on the Strip. Hey, did you catch my act at Caesars'?"

"Yeah, you played Clementine. Key of C. *Oh my Darlin, Oh my Darlin.* The crowd loved it, we heard. Better than Sinatra. They gave you a one-year contract. Induced you to give up medicine. Break a leg."

We appreciated each other's taste in Roots music, and made great fun out of how it's not exactly box office at the big venues. We tended to act haughty, disdainful even, of the popular genres. Not that folk isn't popular, it is to a certain extent. But it's not lucrative. Not even close. Our music tends to get squeezed into remote places, like Gilligan's party room.

The room filled early. Of course 'filled' is relative. About fifty folding chairs arranged in five rows. We rarely had standees.

"Who's your friend?" asked one of the regulars.

"Guys, this is Barbara Wilson. She works with me at the hospital, and has recently taken up ukulele. And she sings."

"Well, you're mighty welcome here Barbara. Feel free to join in."

"Thank you," she said. "I think I'll sit in the audience."

There are two key ingredients to a good jam session: compatible players who keep up with each other, and audience participation for the singing. Gilligan learned early on that the best way to get audience involvement is to show the lyrics as each song is played. Most people who come to these sessions know the melodies, but not the words. So he went high tech with laptop software and equipment that projects lyrics on the wall. Some would say this technology is anti-folk, but that's nonsense. Anything that engages the audience is worthwhile.

The lyrics come with chord notation, which is also helpful to us if we forget some passage. An assistant handles the projection. The order of songs played doesn't matter; any song can be quickly selected and displayed on the wall. Gilligan's laptop holds some 600 songs.

We tuned and began strumming. The audience was a mix of old and young, with a couple of small kids running around. Gilligan welcomed the audience, then looked at his assembled players.

"OK, who wants to go first?" by which he meant who wants to pick the first song.

"Why don't we start with *Down in the Valley*," I said. "Key of G." The song lyrics flashed on the rear wall (chords omitted here), and we began playing.

Down in the valley
Valley so low
Hang your head over
Hear the wind blow

Hear the wind blow, love
Hear the wind blow
Hang your head over
Hear the wind blow

Barbara was tentative. She had not sung in public in years. However, most of the audience warmed up quickly, and sang robustly. Next we did *House of the Rising Sun*, followed by *Charlie and the MTA*.

Outside the bedroom there is no greater pleasure than making music. I love classical, some opera, and Broadway show tunes, but can't play or sing those genres with any authority; I can only be a listener. With folk music I am a participant and that is all the difference in the world to me.

The next song was *Simple Gifts*. Occasionally John would give a little intro, as he did with our second song. "*Simple Gifts* is a traditional Shaker hymn, written in 1848 by one Joseph Brackett," he told the audience, "but virtually unknown outside of the Shaker sect until the mid-1940s. And what changed back then?" he asked.

"*Appalachian Spring*," said a guy in the audience.

"Right. Aaron Copeland's music for the ballet *Appalachian Spring*, first produced in 1944, which I'm sure you've all heard at one time or other. Copeland used the simple Shaker tune to great effect in his music. In fact, eye-watering effect. Please, sing along. Let's play."

'Tis the gift to be simple, 'tis the gift to be free
'Tis the gift to come down where we ought to be,
And when we find ourselves in the place just right,
'Twill be in the valley of love and delight.

When true simplicity is gained,
To bow and to bend we shan't be ashamed,
To turn, turn will be our delight,
Till by turning, turning we come 'round right.

The singing energized Barbara, and she became more animated with each song. We played Pete Seeger's *If I Had a Hammer* and *Little Boxes*, Leonard Cohen's *Hallelujah*, and the depression-era *You Are My Sunshine*. At the conclusion of *Sunshine* I made eye contact with Barbara and mouthed 'I love you.' In Barbara fashion she pointed to herself and mouthed back, "Who, me?" She was having a good time, but had not yet picked up her ukulele. During the break, I said,

"How 'bout Clementine?"

"How 'bout it? The girl drowned."

"You can do it, want to try?"

I can't go up there."

"You don't have to. Strum it from your seat. We'll do it next. Trust me, no one will hear you but yourself."

"I'll try."

After the break I announced *Clementine* as the next song and began strumming the chords. The familiar lyrics flashed on the wall.

> In a cavern, in a canyon,
> Excavating for a mine,
> Dwelt a miner, forty-niner,
> And his daughter Clementine

> Oh my darling, oh my darling
> Oh my darling Clementine
> Thou art lost and gone forever,
> Dreadful sorry, Clementine.

More stanzas followed. As ever, Clementine drowns in the foaming brine. The miner is forlorn, until "I kissed her sister." (The song was written as satire, turns out.) Barbara strummed the few simple chords, expertly I thought. However, as the ukulele is no match for the guitar she did not stand out. No matter. The audience sang, Barbara joined in, and I felt proud of her effort.

The rest of the evening we took audience requests. I hoped Barbara would continue her strumming. The very next song was a winner: *Buffalo Gals (Won't You Come Out Tonight)*.

> As I was walking down the street,
> Down the street, down the street,
> A pretty little gal I chanced to meet,
> Oh, she was fair to see.

Buffalo gals, won't you come out tonight?
Come out tonight, Come out tonight?
Buffalo gals, won't you come out tonight,
And dance by the light of the moon.

The crowd loved it. Barbara sang and strummed. Afterwards two people sitting next to her stood up and applauded – her! She blushed. We
played another ten songs, then called it a night. There would be more
jam sessions to come and Barbara would improve. Just another mutual
interest to hold us together.

CHAPTER 14

———◆———

CARL'S LAWYER WORKED DOWNTOWN, IN one of the many low-rise office buildings around Freemont Street. The sign on the door said Dworkin, Dworkin and Heinz. My appointment was with Harold Dworkin, one of the founding brothers.

Think downtown lawyer and you probably conjure up a guy in a suit, straight arrow, careful talker. Not Dworkin. He could have played a mobster on the Sopranos. Built like a truck, he wore a yellow tie half unknotted, bright pink shirt unbuttoned at the top, with a neat white handkerchief in the left pocket. He sported thick glasses and a crew cut. I would not want to meet up with him in one of those dark alleys.

By now I was seeing everyone as a TV character. Gabe the hustling cable network exec. Carl, the smoothie blackjack boss. Dr. Billington, the corporate CEO. Dworkin, the mobster. Barbara, the innocent sweetie who deserves the good guy. Me, the good guy of course.

"So Carl Collins referred you?"

"Yes, sir."

"Call me Harold. I'll call you Joshua, if you don't mind. I got your contract, and the check for $2000 as retainer. The retainer's just so we can sit and talk business, and I know you're serious. Believe it or not, a lot of people want to BS with you, then decide they don't need a lawyer."

I sensed this guy was all business, but then he proceeded to talk about *himself* for ten minutes. I was glad not to be paying by the minute. He hailed originally from Boston, went to Harvard Law. Moved to Vegas thirty years ago. Happily married. Two kids, four grandkids. Plays golf, too. Has a ten handicap, despite his bulk. Loves Vegas. Said I made the right decision to move here. Finally, he got down to the issue at hand – my potential contract with Triple X-Las Vegas.

"How well do you know Gabe Stein?"

"Not well. Met him twice. Carl knows him much better."

"And so you want to invest 100,000 dollars in this new cable show?

"It seems so."

"Umm. And you're a doctor?

"Yes."

"What kind of doctor?"

"Emergency Medicine. At Memorial."

"Carl told me a little about the show you and Gabe plan to produce, but just explain to me, a summary. It's a variety show, I understand."

I outlined the acts Gabe and I had discussed, including the Biggest Loser contest. He wasn't surprised or disgusted, just said, "Well, that sounds like Gabe and Triple X-Las Vegas." He thought for a moment.

"Joshua, it's obvious to me you're a nice guy, and frankly, you came to the right lawyer for doing business with Gabe. I'll be honest, it's a gamble, though you could make a lot of money in this venture. However, if you want to quit, back out now, I'm not going to cash your check. I've spent most of the time talking about myself anyway, so let me know if you still want to proceed. If you do, I'll cash your check and represent you, and you won't be sorry. With me at least. Can't say how this venture will work out."

I felt a little foolish. I was there in his office, I wanted to make the investment, but this older, wiser guy was giving me an out, and it wouldn't cost me a dime.

"No, Harold, I think I'm in it. I can afford to lose the money, but obviously my goal is to make some."

"OK. Good. Let's begin, then. The contract is a pile of garbage. Gabe knows it's unworkable, but he always starts with garbage, then we get things ironed out. You read it?"

"Well, yes, but it's all legalese."

"I made a little list. First, he didn't specify *when* you would be paid. He could take a year or a century with this contract. Second, he doesn't specify accounting methods or guarantee you access to the books on this specific show. He has to keep legit records for the IRS, and in fact he does, but he doesn't specify you have full access. As co-producer you have a right to see the full accounting. Otherwise, he could say the show made money, lost money, whatever. What are you going to do? Third, he has an indemnity clause. He wants *you* to indemnify *him* for any lawsuits arising out of this show."

"He does?"

"Yeah, standard legal prose. It's right here," and he pointed to Section 18c. "The undersigned will indemnify XXX-Las Vegas for any losses due to legal or contract disputes arising out of *Consenting Adults Only*." I had skimmed over that part.

"Wow," I muttered. "Missed that."

"There's other things. I'll fix them. Carl owns most of the network, and stands to benefit the most from any success. As co-producer of just one of Triple X's offerings, the most you should be at risk for is your 100,000 dollar investment. Nothing more."

"Well, I certainly agree."

"Now the good news," said Harold.

"OK. I'm listening."

"He's a straight shooter and won't actively try to cheat you. But he will passively mess with you, if you sign a piece of garbage like this. If the contract lets him get away with something, he'll more than likely try it. He looks for every angle of advantage. But when I present him with a real contract he'll sign it like a pussy cat. And he'll honor it. That's the way he does business. You'll be as legally well-protected as anyone who invests in an untested, untried, disgusting cable porn show can be. No, Gabe Stein is not your biggest concern."

"What is?"

"The show itself. It's a piece of crap." Harold laughed so hard at his punchline, he started coughing.

Everyone in this town seemed to be a comedian.

———

Harold had a new contract to me the following week. All the offensive stuff was eliminated. I approved and he sent it on to Gabe's lawyer. As Dworkin predicted, Gabe signed it without objection. I then issued a banker's check to XXX-Las Vegas for $100,000. We were on our way. The first show was tentatively scheduled in six weeks, the end of January.

CHAPTER 15

———

CHRISTMAS SEASON WAS UPON US, and what with my own night-day schedule, the first post-contract meeting we could arrange was December 27. I was now co-producer and so Gabe wanted me involved. I was also liaison to Jack, who was liaison to the women who would compete for Biggest Loser, bathroom version. That was to be the contest theme. Since you can't copyright a show name, Gabe figured it would attract more people already in love with the regular TV show.

At this meeting I also met Brendan McKnight, the man Gabe hired as host or emcee. He had worked for Gabe before on a now-defunct porn show, the one Gabe referred to at our first meeting. Brendan is a few years older than me. He has a fine, deep voice and chiseled face good for TV. Of course I knew nothing about him, not even what he did for a living when not emceeing one of Triple X's rare live shows.

Anyway, we laid out the first variety show, which I got to name. Gabe wanted to call it The Biggest Loser Variety Show. That sounded lame to me because only part of the show was about weight reduction, and the title made it sound like the other actors were losers.

"You have a better name?"

"Let me think," I said. "How about 'The Triple X Variety Hour'?"

Gabe guffawed. "Too, too generic. Sounds like Ed Sullivan. Do you know who he was?"

I actually did, because his variety hour in the 50s and 60s catapulted both Elvis and the Beatles to nationwide fame. Documentaries on the rise of Elvis and the Beatles always mentioned Sullivan. "Of course," I said.

"Well, I'm not doing Ed Sullivan. This is not a family show."

"OK, OK, I get that." Then it hit me. "What's the common theme here, Gabe?"

"Fucking? Sex?"

"No, no. People doing their own thing, voluntarily. I know some out there call it porn, but it's just people doing their own thing, without harming anyone else. Consenting adults. That's it! *Consenting Adults Only.*" He liked it. We had our name.

Looking back, the title was about my only contribution to birthing the show. Gabe presented a tentative format for the first one, a full 90 minutes.

Part 1
0:00 – 0:02 Introduce new show. Welcome to XXX-Las Vegas, etc. Rules: No video or photography in audience. Remind audience to please fill questionnaire before leaving, etc.
0:02 – 0:12 Three Biggest Loser contestants introduced. They will wear Bikinis; ck re: topless? Weighing of contestants. Contestants retreat to studio rear, to use bathrooms.
0:12 – 0:20 Sex Act #1; TBD
0:20 – 0:28 Home Video #1; TBD
0:28 – 0:30 – Ad - Sex toy demonstration

Part 2
0:30 – 0:40 - Sex Act #2; TBD
0:40 – 0:45 - Home Video #2; TBD
0:45 – 0:50 – Ad - Sex toy demonstration

<u>Part 3</u>
0:50 – 0:60 – Sex Act #3; TBD
0:60 – 0:70 - Home Video #3; TBD
0:70 – 0:78 - Return of Biggest Loser contestants. Each woman is weighed, winner announced and she is interviewed. Emphasize her preparation for show, what she ate and drank during the day, etc.
0:78 – 0:80 – Ad – Sex toy demonstration
0:80 – 0:84 - Audience votes on best Home Video
0:84 – 0:88 - Audience votes on best Live Sex Act
0:88 – 0:90 - Final Words; announce the next show will be in one week

Consenting Adults Only would be followed by the usual porn fare, turning into gay and lesbian videos around 1 am. I asked about the show's length.

"Anything longer than 90 minutes and the audience needs a bathroom break," said Gabe. "You lose momentum. Anything shorter and they feel they wasted their time driving out here. Ninety minutes is ideal."

I also asked what the "Sex Acts" would be but was brushed aside with "standard stuff, nothing we haven't done before. We have some options. That's why it's all listed as TBD. To be determined."

CHAPTER 16

———

V<small>ISITORS AT THE BIGGEST</small> V<small>EGAS</small> hotels are routinely solicited for live events, many for free. The free ones are often a scam of some sort, to sell real estate or something else you didn't come to Vegas for. You get there and they hold you captive for two hours. However, new, legitimate shows, frequently also give away tickets to fill seats, or foster audience word-of-mouth publicity. Savvy visitors take the tickets, then do an investigation on their smart phone. God help the freebie that is trashed in social media.

Gabe Stein arranged for distribution of over 3000 colorful flyers -- "invitations for tickets" -- in the three days before the first show. In each corner of the flyer a bikini-clad model posed seductively. The flyers read:

XXX-Las Vegas
What You Won't See on Regular Cable

XXX-Las Vegas invites you to a new Cable show, *Consenting Adults Only*, CAO will feature acts and activities not seen live anywhere else in Las Vegas. Check us out at www.XXX-LasVegas, for a listing of our popular cable programs. To attend our new cable show as part of a live audience, please call 702 --- ----. We will then send you an e-mail ticket, which you must present on arrival (paper or smart phone is acceptable).

When you call you will NOT be asked for any other identifying information or your credit card. The show is free.

NOTE: Please be aware. Some of these acts and activities deal with normal heterosexual and bodily functions, and may be offensive. Our goal is not to offend but to entertain. Men and women 21 and over are welcome. Expect to spend about 2 hours at the location you will be given, but you may of course leave anytime. Upon exiting you will be asked to fill out a brief and anonymous audience questionnaire. Our audience will be limited to the first 200 who call for tickets.

You can't distribute anything in the hotel itself or even on the premises, so people were targeted as they exited or approached the properties. I thought the flyer was honest and straightforward. If you come to Las Vegas and get handed a flyer like this, you'd be an idiot to think the show is *Mary Poppins*. No one who showed up should be shocked by the "acts and activities."

I asked Stein why he didn't put an ad in the paper. He said the flyer distributors were trained to look for male and female high-end tourists. An ad in the paper was more likely to attract low-end, including Vegas's share of local perverts.

Overall, pretty good marketing, I thought.

———◆———

In early January, after a long hospital day, I arrived home to a surprise. Barbara said there was a small package in the mail. I didn't remember ordering anything. The return address was a PO Box number in Beaverton, OR. I knew no one in Oregon.

I opened it and inside found a bottle of pills and a glossy one-page brochure. "Congratulations on ordering Erecto Pills," it read, followed by instructions on how to use them. They were from a company called

"Fix-it-UP." Of course I never ordered anything from Fix-it-UP or any other outfit peddling pills for sexual dysfunction. How did I get on their mailing list? I had a good idea, but told Barbara otherwise.

"I have no idea. Must be they got my name from a Vegas doctors' list, hoping I'll tell my patients about them."

"Well, you certainly don't need them," she deadpanned.

In bed I decided to level with Barbara. I am not good at holding secrets and too many were piling up. I didn't want them to come out later, lest she think I was holding back or being deceptive. So I told her about the apartment trashing and the brief phone call from Judy. I said I was pretty certain the Fix-it-Up package was Judy's idea, hoping to put a wrench in our relationship, and that I would not be surprised if we heard more from her. I followed this with kisses and expressions of love and how we seemed destined to end up husband and wife.

"But I'm not Jewish," she said, knowing of course it made no difference whatever. We had discussed this before. She was just being playful.

"Yes," I said, "and I'm not Christian. So we're even."

Then she began to cry.

"Barb, it's OK. It's just you and me. No need to cry."

"I guess I have my own little secret. One I've kept from you."

I shuddered. Was she married after all? With children somewhere? "Oh?"

"She burst into tears.

"Oh my God, Barbara, what's the matter?"

She could not talk for crying. I asked no more. I knew she would tell me her secret when the crying stopped.

She finally subsided. "It's OK, Barbara. It's OK. You can tell me when you're ready. There's no rush."

"I had an abortion."

"What? When?"

"A year after I arrived in Vegas. I lied a little about Trader John's Saloon. No, that's not true, Josh. I lied a lot about the place. It was a cesspool. It was superficial, the girls were all dreamers and I was too, initially. Yeah, there is a pole dancers' union, but it only protects your basic wage, not your morals. Girls get propositioned a lot and you have to be a saint to keep from getting rolled over by the high rollers. You think men are going to just throw money at you and not expect something in return? So every night it was a struggle. Some girls survived, some didn't. I stayed at it because the money was good and I was smart enough to keep my perspective."

"What happened?"

She hesitated. "I've got to sit up. Wait a minute." She propped herself up on pillows. I joined her in the sitting position. We held hands, which seemed oddly appropriate at just that moment.

"Are you sure you still want to tell me?"

"Now that I've started, yes. I went out with one guy who came to the show a couple of times and seemed genuinely interested in me. I went out with him after his second visit. He had a lot of money. Told me he was a hedge fund trader in New York, here on business. He had a limousine and a driver. We visited a couple of nightclubs. And here's the crazy thing. The guy was interesting, a very rich businessman with a sense of humor. I mean, we laughed a lot, and I sort of grew to like him."

"Just the one date?"

"Just one. His limousine, you can imagine, has a spacious back seat. We kissed, he fondled, I pushed his hands away a few times. I said no, not now, please, and resisted in a way a gentleman would respect. Then he turned brutish. I had had a few drinks, but was not drunk. He wouldn't take no for an answer. His driver kept driving, didn't act like anything was amiss, though I was clearly resisting him. I imagine this had been played out before in this guy's limos. Long story short, he raped me in the back seat. He was strong and I couldn't stop him."

She began crying, softly. Now sitting seemed awkward. I held her around the waist and we slid back to a flat position.

"I'm so sorry, Barbara."

"Oh, Josh, hold me, please." Her sobbing increased.

Tears welled up in my eyes. I wiped them away with the blanket. I waited a minute, until her crying ceased.

"Are you OK?"

"Yes. I'm sorry I didn't tell you."

"Are you kidding? You shouldn't be sorry at all. Did you file charges?"

"Hardly. He would have claimed it was consensual, and his driver would have testified on his behalf, I'm sure. I cried afterwards like a baby, just like now. He took me home and I never saw him again at the Saloon."

"And you got pregnant?"

"Yes. Three weeks later, no period. Like an idiot, I wasn't taking the pill then. I had just been accepted to nursing school. The last thing I needed was a baby, without a father. I had the abortion at eight weeks. I've felt guilty about it ever since. No one knows but Irene, and she swore she'll never tell. Not even Carl knows. Now you know. I can't hide it any longer. I will feel forever feel guilty for murdering my unborn child."

"I am so sorry," I repeated. There is little solace for a woman so bereaved. I held her tight. "Barbara, you'll have more children. If I have anything to do with it."

"I wanted to tell you before, but couldn't. Well, now you know. I'm glad it's off my chest." She sobbed, softly this time.

I kissed her gently. At least I had an answer about relationships after she moved to Vegas. Was there more? I pulled myself up on one elbow and asked: "There's nothing more? No more deep, deep, dark, dark secrets you want to tell me? Before or after coming to Vegas?"

There was no immediate answer, not a good sign.

"Well?"

"Not tonight."

"Not tonight? What's that supposed to mean?"

"Josh, I had some issues early on that I'd rather not go into. Please, another time. I love you and what's past is past. I've only been pregnant once in my life, so there's no orphanage out there holding Barbara's kid. I know that's what you're thinking, right?"

"Actually, the thought crossed my mind. So an unhappy affair as a teenager, something like that?"

"OK, something like that."

"Or pre-teen?" I was getting nosy, but why not? I was living with her, planned to marry her, and had a right to know these things.

"Please don't Josh, PLEASE. Not tonight. Another time, OK?"

"OK, OK." I figured when the time came she would tell me. At least, thank goodness, there was no hidden child.

"How about with you?" she asked.

"What?"

"Any deep dark secrets? Like maybe you *were* married to Judy at one time, but forgot?"

I laughed. "Nothing more. No more secrets. You know it all."

"Pinky swear?"

She held out up her little finger, left hand. I enclosed it with the little finger of my right hand. "Pinky swear."

CHAPTER 17

———

XXX-LAS VEGAS WAS LOCATED IN a stand-alone, single-story building, part of a commercial park in the suburbs. I estimated the floor space at about 10,000 square feet. It had the type of interior space that can be modified to suit just about any tenant's needs. I learned Gabe was in his third year of a ten-year lease. A small sign on the lawn read "XXX-Las Vegas." For all anyone could tell, the business inside could be tic-tac-toe.

The auditorium was small and cozy, with stadium seats ending at a floor-level stage. On either side of the stage sat two large projection TVs, each capable of showing whatever the videographers shoot. This technique is used in many venues, most famously at Grand Ole Opry in Nashville. There, it is used to good effect to show close ups of country singers' faces, which can be difficult to see from the far away seats. At Triple X the screens made it easy for the audience to see the sex close up, if they wish. What was on the screens was also what the cable and internet audiences viewed in their homes.

I didn't know what to expect when I arrived, an hour before show time. Gabe gave me a brief tour of the building, then introduced me to several people who would appear on the first show. They were ensconced in what TV people call the Green Room, a holding area for guests. Thankfully, during introductions he did not call me "doctor."

In the Green Room I met three young couples, the live "TBD" sex acts. The three female weight loss contestants were in a separate area, preparing for their contest with some last-minute drinking and eating.

"So you're the co-producer" said one of the guys, named Jerry. Jerry was with Juniper, his girlfriend.

"Yes, I'm new to this business." Jerry didn't ask what my old business was.

"Well, we've worked with Gabe before. Great channel, he has."

"You're from Las Vegas?" I asked.

"No, me and Juniper came over from LA. Did you see an RV parked out front?"

"Yes. Yours?"

"Our home away from home."

"Actually, Joshua," said Juniper, in corrective mode, "it's our home *at* home. We live in the Valley, in an RV park. Keeps us mobile, we go wherever the jobs are."

"So what do you do in LA?" I asked, though I sort of knew the answer already.

"Same," said Jerry, "but business is slowing down there, with the ever-present AIDS scare. That's all you hear. The industry isn't what it used to be. So we travel around. How'd you get connected with Gabe?"

"Mutual friend, who knew Gabe. He works at the Argonaut."

"Who is it? We know lots of Gabe's old friends."

"Guy named Carl Collins."

"You know Carl?" said Jerry.

"Yes. He's a friend." I didn't add, 'of a friend'.

"Carl used to work with us in the Valley! Haven't seen him in a few years. What's he doing at the Argonaut?"

"He's a blackjack dealer. Actually, he's head of several blackjack tables. He's the pit boss."

"I'll be damned," said Jerry. "Moving up in the world. Got out of the porn business. Always wondered what happened to him."

I marveled at the situation: a Jewish guy from the Midwest talking pornography geography in Las Vegas.

———

The first show started on time, with Brendan the emcee. I watched from one of the stage wings. Brendan's voice projected well; I could see why Gabe chose him.

"These three lovely women will compete tonight in Vegas's own version of the Biggest Loser. Are you ready, ladies?"

The women nodded yes, no doubt counting the grand each would receive for going to the bathroom.

"Number one, what is your name please, and where are you from?"

"Holly, from Phoenix."

"And you living in Vegas now?"

"Yes, for about six months."

"Well OK, Holly. Welcome to Vegas and welcome to Triple X."

During this introduction the two black-clad videographers did their thing, showing full frontal and rear images, with the occasional close up of breasts and buttocks. There was more purpose in this than titillation. It was to give time for internet subscribers to bet on the contestants.

"Number two, what is your name and where are you from?"

"Ginger, I'm from right here in Las Vegas." More frontal and rear images.

"That's quite some bikini, Ginger. Who's the guy on the front, the one lying on a beach chair?"

"That's my boyfriend."

"Does he know you put his picture right in front, between your legs and below your belly button?"

"Yes. It was his idea. That's where he wants to be."

The audience laughed. Gabe stood close by and I heard him say, to no one in particular, "This is great."

"And, last but not least, number three."

"Maryann, from Vegas also."

"Maryann, is this your first time on cable television?"

"Yes." She giggled and gave a light shoulder shrug, which anyone watching would infer as 'Oh my I can't believe I'm doing this'.

"Well, don't be nervous. You gals are great, and we thank you for appearing on *Consenting Adults Only*. Now, we've asked our audience to write down what they think each of you weighs, bikini included. We're going to take a short commercial break, and when we return I'll weigh you. Then you will go to your dressing rooms and return in about an hour."

The screens then showed a picture of all three women side by side. On your computer you would see a place to enter four numbers for each woman, with a decimal fraction. You entered your weight guess– e.g., 343.6 -- and if you hit the weight on the nose, you won. If your guess was within a pound you got your money back, an added incentive to bet. To enter the contest you pre-paid five dollars.

After the commercial break -- some type of sex toy guaranteed to "make her want more" -- Brendan asked the women to step on the scale, one at a time. Their digital weights popped onto the video screen.

"Here we go, number one. 327.7 pounds! How many in the audience got within five pounds?" Several hands went up. "Within one pound?" One hand up. "On the nose?" The one hand went down. This scene was repeated for the other two contestants.

"We have our weights," said Brendan, and he repeated the numbers. "Are you ready, audience?"

They responded in unison: "Yes!"

"OK, gals, go do your thing. You will be re-weighed in about an hour. So relax." The audience tittered.

Jack had delivered. The women were large but not unattractive. They all wore bikinis, thankfully. Negotiations to appear naked had gone nowhere. Even so, very little was hidden by the two-piece suits.

Their breasts were pendulous, their thighs enormous, their buttocks protuberant. If you saw them on a beach you would probably look just once.

I had one other thought. Unlike the men at Joe's Plumbing Supplies, who wore big boxer shorts and had to be checked to rule out lead-weight jock straps, there was no way these women could hide anything of the sort.

———

The rest of the show was what most people would call porn, and was divided into two categories: things men and women do to each other, live, on stage; and home videos. The first category was Triple X's specialty. As with Irene's and Carl's video, the cameramen took angled shots, close ups and the occasional full view. In addition, the lighting guy darkened the stage, then used selective spotlights to highlight the main activity. From an artistic expression point of view it was well done. The details are not necessary to recount, but I learned later there was betting involved over these acts. Exactly what the metric was, I wasn't sure. I should also mention a few people did leave after the first sex act. Didn't they read the flyer?

Home videos were made by real people in unreal circumstances. The only requirement was the video had to show sex between a man and a woman, and *no bedroom scenes.* Triple X was looking for creativity. The winner, voted on by the live audience, would get $1000.

My thought after seeing the first home video: better than *America's Funniest Videos.* I mean, screwing while sky-diving? The man and woman were assembled half-naked in some type of parachute-equipped harness. They fell out of the plane with a third guy, who shot the video; he was also there, it seemed, to remind the romancing couple to "open your parachutes."

The video was jerky and you couldn't really tell if they did it or not. All you saw were twisting, naked behinds. During the free fall, the audience laughed, which was entirely appropriate. It was funny. When the couple landed, still alive, the audience cheered. There surely is some category where this couple would win first prize (stupidest sky diving stunt?), but not in our contest.

The second home video was the water skiing couple. The videographer was in a speed boat right next to the skiers. This couple was so good, they could have auditioned for Cirque du Soleil and been hired on the spot. I mean, they did it on skis, going thirty miles an hour. At least he penetrated, but I don't think either came to climax. As they unwound on their respective skis, each took a naked bow. Very impressive. The audience cheered them as well.

The third video featured a zip line duo. The background was lush, probably some Central American jungle. She goes out on a zip line and gets stuck. The guy on the platform from where she started has a large mustache and looks like Super Mario. "Give me a minute," he yells out to her, "I'll rescue you." "Oh, thank you, kind sir," she yells back, while her eyelids flutter.

He takes off his pants, puts on the harness and zips after her. He gets behind her and starts fondling. She likes it, gets in the mood. One guy on each of the two platforms that connect the zip line shoot video of the rescue, so you get to see front and back images. Next thing you know Super Mario enters her from behind and she pretends a climax; it certainly seemed fake to me. There is music and the words "Zip Line Heaven" appear on the screen. Creative, and cute, but for my money didn't hold a candle to the water skiing duo.

Gabe had a library of these videos, and planned to show the best ones on the remaining five shows. The ones I saw during the first show were a hoot.

———

Consenting Adults Only, Week One, was a success. Ticket requests for Week Two began the next day and remained steady throughout the week. Whether you liked the content or not, it was a legitimate show and delivered as promised. Gabe told me afterwards that a full accounting of the show, including all the on-line betting, would take several weeks. I had no reason to doubt him, and looked forward to the next show and my future profits.

CHAPTER 18

I WAS GLAD TO GET back to the hospital. XXX-Las Vegas was a kinky diversion, a glimpse into the world of sex workers and elimination contests and cable television, but medicine is where I belonged. Many people would look askance at someone in Gabe's business, no matter how legitimate or lucrative. But if you're in the medical field you are solid, respectable. It felt good and safe to work in the Emergency Department.

Two days after the first show, I received a 10 x 13 inch brown envelope, with no return address. It arrived to my mail box at the hospital. Inside I found a four-page letter, typed single-spaced, from Judy. It began:

> Dear Josh,
> I want to explain my reason for writing you this long letter. Please read it to the end, and I think you will have a better understanding of my situation.

The letter went downhill from there. I found it chilling, with its obsession over events real and imagined, alternation of child-like sweetness and grown-up anger, and veiled threats. This was the first time I realized – fully realized – Judy was a sick woman, and I was a focus of her illness. I will quote just a few paragraphs here, to provide a flavor of her madness.

...You said "the relationship is over for now." I remember those words well. They came to me clearly when I drove back to Los Angeles. Over for now means not forever, so enough time has passed, don't you think, that over for now has passed, and now is the time? Don't you agree that now is passed and now is the time? I have thought this through clearly, and analyzed it, and I am certain that now is over and now is the time. Don't you agree?

...I do see a problem of what to do with the bitch. I am not suggesting anything serious happen to her. I would not want that, it would be unkind, yes it would. I know she works in your hospital and perhaps you can find her another job in another hospital and not in your bedroom? Don't you think? I would really like you to work on this, and the sooner the better. It would make the most sense if you found her another job not in your hospital and not in your bedroom. You can do this Josh. You must do this.

...I can't come to Las Vegas right now but you can come to Los Angeles. We have better weather in Los Angeles, and you could meet me here. Another thing, as if you didn't know, we have angels! That's why we're the City of Angels. But call first, I don't want to be embarrassed by your coming in unannounced (hah! hah!). You have my phone number my number has not changed and I know yours has.

...I want you to think of all these things and get back to me as soon as possible. I think this correspondence is a good thing and I am so glad I thought of it. I do want to see you again and know you must want the same. Call me when you get this and we can discuss us further.

After two more "call me" paragraphs she ended,

With much love that you should return, you really, really should. Judy.

Her letter suggested she might be psychotic. But how could she work as a doctor if she was truly psychotic? Some other psychiatric diagnosis, perhaps. "Crazed Lover" for sure, but the term isn't in the Diagnostic and Statistical Manual of Mental Disorders, the bible of psychiatric diagnoses.

Was she even under psychiatric care? On one hand I wanted to get her help. On the other hand, I wanted nothing to do with her, certainly not send any false signal to suggest we should get back together. Why did I not see any of this when we were dating? She became demanding during our relationship, but I didn't think at the time she was *crazy*. Did my breaking up with her trigger a latent condition?

The only rational course for me was to do nothing, and hope her illness would be discovered by others and she would come under treatment. And leave me alone.

Her letter presented one other conundrum. I promised Barbara no secrets. I would break that promise now. She would never see this letter. It was way too scary. At the same time I felt it should preserved, as evidence of some kind I might need or want one day. I decided to put it in a safe deposit box at the bank. But first I would show it to a colleague at the hospital.

———————

Working in the ED you get to meet most of the medical staff, either because they come down to see patients or you have to call them about an admission. Psychiatry is different; all admissions are handled directly by the Psychiatry department. The ED staff only gets involved if a patient has to be "medically cleared" for admission to Psychiatry. Still, I got to know the staff psychiatrists, from frequent phone conversations, and meeting them in the doctors' lounge and at occasional staff parties.

In this way I came to know Dr. Rose Sobel, a seasoned psychiatrist in her early 50s. Jewish doctors in Vegas tend to gravitate toward each other, but she was also more approachable than most of her colleagues. I never felt like she was "analyzing" me, which is not the case with some other psychiatrists. So I felt comfortable calling her about the letter. I just wanted her opinion. To my delight, she seemed interested, especially given that Judy is a physician. We agreed to meet for lunch in the hospital cafeteria the next day.

———

Dr. Sobel and I found a table with reasonable privacy and sat down to talk and eat our salads.

"Don't show me the letter just yet, Josh. First, just tell me some background about her."

"Well, we first met in medical school, but didn't date then."

"So in medical school you didn't find anything unusual?"

"No, but I didn't have much contact with her. She married this fellow student and I think she lived with him her senior year, so we had no more than a student-student relationship. She's a B and I'm an L in the alphabet, so we weren't even in the same sections together. I remember talking with her once at a Jewish social event and thinking she was attractive, but she was already hooked up then. Why would I suspect she was nutso? Besides, what do we know in medical school anyway? When did you get interested in psychiatry?"

"From day one," Dr. Sobel said. "I always knew that's what I wanted to do. I read Freud in high school."

"Yeah, well you were precocious. My psych rotation wasn't very psycho-analytical, so Freud was kind of de-emphasized. Ironically, one thing recommended was the movie *Fatal Attraction*. Ever see it?"

"Yes. I remember it as pretty scary."

"Well, the Glenn Close character, Alex Forrest, that's who Judy reminds me of."

"Now. But you told me on the phone you dated her for six months."

The loud speaker blared "Code Blue, 3 East. Code Blue, 3 East." Four residents scurried from their tables and ran out of the cafeteria. In cardiac arrest seconds count. Thankfully it wasn't a patient in the ED, or I would have been the one scurrying. My ED colleague had me covered for routine patients.

"I remember those codes. I used to run like that." Dr. Sobel said.

"You did a medicine internship?"

"Oh, yes. A year of internal medicine. It was valuable training for psychiatry. Too many shrinks know no medicine, none at all. Where were we?"

"I had dated her for six months."

"Oh, yes. For six months. So you must have learned something."

"It was off and on. Don't forget, she lives in Los Angeles."

"But she must have told you something about her background, her family."

"Actually, she did, now that I think about it. I remember she told me her father was an alcoholic and he was abusive to her mother. Her parents were divorced and there'd been no contact with her dad for years. She had a miserable childhood, but after a while we didn't talk about our pasts. They were different, and I felt awkward comparing childhoods. Anyway, when she became more demanding and controlling, I didn't make any connection between her behavior and her childhood. I guess that's why I'm not in psychiatry."

"Give me an example of how she became more demanding."

"OK. I was once at her apartment in LA. I drove in on a Friday night, with plans to return here Sunday morning. I had the weekend off but a lot of work to do before returning to work on Monday, and wanted to get back early. Well, she went ballistic. 'Why are you leaving so early, I made plans to go to the beach on Sunday, you've got to go with me, don't walk out on me'. She carried on like a child. I honestly had the impression she might hurt herself if I didn't adhere to her schedule. So I stayed and drove back Sunday night. It was an uncomfortable weekend."

"And how did you break up?"

I recounted the whole story, of how Judy let herself in the night I slept with Barbara, how Barbara was wearing only my shirt when she walked into the living room, and that Judy told Barbara we were married. I told her about Judy's bras and panties in the bedroom dresser, and then how Barbara stormed out of the apartment.

"Sounds like you were in a sticky situation," she said.

"That's an understatement. For a moment I felt like I was in a sit-com. The audience might be laughing but trust me, I wasn't."

"I'm just trying to picture it. There you are, standing in your own apartment with two women, one nude except for a shirt, the other fully dressed, just arrived from LA. You've been intimate with both, and both want to keep you. You are wary of the old girlfriend Judy and clearly like the new girlfriend Barbara. So my question is, why didn't you just ask Judy to return to Los Angeles, instead of letting Barbara leave?"

"Honestly, Rose, events went so fast, before I knew it Barbara was gone. And then, before I knew it, I was back in bed with Judy. I was afraid of her, at least in her lust-for-Joshua mood. The next morning, when she was in a calmer mood, I officially severed our relationship."

"But you had sex with Judy? I find that a little hard to believe, considering the circumstances."

I squirmed a bit. Our conversation was not just between two doctors, but between a man and a woman. I felt uncomfortable recounting what we actually did in bed. To her credit she sensed my discomfort.

"Don't be embarrassed. I'm not trying to pry into your bedroom activities. But somehow you satisfied her lust?"

"Yes, that's fair to say. I satisfied her."

"And then you broke up with her?"

"The next morning."

"How'd she take it?"

"Not well, but she didn't give any hint of revenge or reprisals. She returned my apartment key and I walked her to her car. I told her I wanted to stay friends, and she sort of agreed. Then she left. Fortunately I was able to get back together with Barbara."

"And what happened afterwards?"

I recounted Judy's trashing my apartment the same day, followed by the phone call and then the Erecto Pills package.

"And her letter was the next thing?"

"Yes, that's when I called you."

"OK," she said, "I think I get the picture. Let me see the letter." I handed it over and she began reading. All I heard for the next several minutes was a subdued ummm, hah, and wow. I continued to work on my salad.

When finished reading she asked, "You're pretty certain she's still working as an ED physician in LA? As far as you know she's functioning?"

"As far as I know, but remember my last contact was when I saw her leave the parking lot. I'm pretty certain she was working then. But I don't know for certain now."

"Well," she said, "first let me make the usual disclaimer. You can't fully diagnose someone from a letter or a second hand history. With that caveat, I think I can give a reasonable assessment."

"I'm all ears."

"She has a borderline personality disorder."

"Not psychotic?"

"Not psychotic, at least not in the traditional sense."

"So this is one of those psychiatric diagnoses I never really understood. Help me out a little."

"The family history, her behavior when you were dating, her actions since you broke up, and this letter – they all fit. She has extremely poor coping skills. Someone who is psychotic might be able to function on medication, but what you've told me and what I've just read are much more consistent with a borderline personality disorder. She's angry, she's frustrated, and she's taking it out on you."

"Rose, I couldn't give you a textbook definition of borderline if my life depended on it. I'd like to check Wikipedia, my go-to source for all things medical. Do you mind?"

"No, not at all. But if I come to your ED in diabetic coma, are you going to look up my treatment on Wikipedia?"

"Nope. But if you come in with a borderline personality disorder, I sure will." We both laughed.

I googled the diagnosis and a web site higher ranked than Wikipedia dealt with psychiatric definitions. I entered the term.

"OK, Rose, this is not Wikipedia, but it seems pretty concise. Want me to read it to you?"

"Please do."

"Borderline personality disorder (BPD) – a psychiatric diagnosis. People with BPD suffer from impaired social skills, marked by a very poor ability to cope with life stressors and also the use of primitive defense mechanisms."

I paused.

"Is that it?" she asked.

"No, there's more. I'm just trying to take in the first part." I continued reading.

"They tend to act impulsively to stressful situations, and often manifest severe mood swings, periods of rage and/or irritability. As result, patients with BPD tend to form poor and unstable interpersonal relationships. They can also manifest both suicidal and homicidal tendencies."

"That's it," I said.

"Well, it's a layman's definition, but fairly accurate," she said.

"Rose, I think you've nailed it. I am most grateful. I have a much better understanding now."

"You're most welcome. Glad to be of service."

"So I guess with this disorder, she could try to kill herself?"

"That is always a possibility."

"Or kill others?"

"That, too, is a possibility."

CHAPTER 19

—◆—

I ARRIVED AN HOUR BEFORE the beginning of *Consenting Adults Only*, Week Two. The hardest part was arranging my ED schedule so I could be there. I just felt the need to be present. Before the first show I had visions of the whole project being a scam, but when the first audience arrived, and the show proved moderately successful, my anxiety evaporated.

In truth, I was fascinated by the show business aspects. Again I see myself as Curious George (or Josh), the monkey willing to poke into anything that looks interesting. Perhaps not a good analogy, since he frequently gets into trouble. But those are kids' books, right?

Gabe was happy with results of the first show, and eager for the second. Whereas we filled only about 150 seats the first time, for the second show we had a full house. "We turned people away," he said.

Many in the audience knew what to expect and were in a good mood. Doors opened an hour before the show.

Thirty minutes before the show Gabe came up to me.

"Bad news."

"Oh?"

"Brendan's not coming."

"Brendan's not coming?"

"He's indisposed. Can't make it."

"Without Brendan, what are we going to do?" There was no backup emcee. "Can't you do it?" I asked.

"With my accent? What do you think?" He really said, "Wit my accent. What do you tink?" I saw his point. Then he looked at me, raising his eyes and chin ever so slightly.

"Oh no, oh no," I said. "I'm not going out there. I'm a doctor, not an emcee."

"We'll cancel the show."

"What do you mean?"

"Just what I said. I'll make an announcement over the PA system. Show canceled. Very sorry, ladies and gentleman. We will resume on further notice. They'll understand enough, even with my accent. They paid nothing, so no refunds. No big deal."

"And reschedule?"

"Cancellation is kiss of death. Word gets out, we may not go on again. Fucking social media. They'll twitter: 'I came, wasted my night. Bastards canceled show with us in audience. Should have gone to see Cirque. Forget Triple X'."

"Will Brendan be back next week?"

"Hope so." Gabe was suspiciously non-committal.

"And if we cancel? My investment?"

"Up in smoke."

I thought back to the contract, which was now almost word for word in my head after Harold's rewrite. There was no guarantee the full six shows would be produced, no mention of refund. Dworkin the lawyer just wanted to make sure I didn't lose more than $100,000. Fair enough. But $100,000 is no small potatoes.

What rankled me is that the first show had been moderately successful. So I saw this as one of those existential, career-defining moments. This stuff happens on Broadway all the time, but then the understudy is primed for the role, eager to step in. I was neither primed nor eager to go on stage. However, I thought I *could* do Brendan's job, so now there was opportunity. But why would I, a respected ED doctor, want to go before a live audience and emcee sex acts and excretion contests? I already told you: my investment and my ego. Where were Barbara, Carl, my parents, to yank me away?

"Gabe, you're saying if I don't take Brendan's place, you might cancel the show permanently?"

"Good possibility. If Brendan can't get back for the next one and I don't find a replacement."

"Then do I get a refund?"

He laughed. "Know what, Josh? *You* have a sense of humor. I like that. Now go break a leg."

———◆———

Of course I would not reveal my real name. In thirty minutes I had to come up with an alias, a point Gabe did not argue. I didn't even want to *look* like Joshua Luvkin, MD. Gabe had an idea. He kept some props in the back, including assorted wigs. I tried several on, found one that changed my relatively close haircut into a mop of unruly hair. In the mirror it was obviously a wig, but didn't look bad. He also found a fake mustache which I put on. *Oh my God! What am I doing?*

Thirty minutes later I was on the stage.

"Good evening. Welcome to XXX-Las Vegas. I am Mel Hopewell, tonight's emcee. You are in for a real entertainment tonight. Let's get started..."

It was not that difficult. I had the list of acts to read from, and since I was familiar with the format from the first show could adlib as necessary. The two video guys were as always consummate professionals, and kept the audience engaged with close ups. From the on-stage TV screens I could tell the lighting was superb.

The Biggest Loser contestants did what they were supposed to: lose weight during the show. The three women were easy to talk to, charming even. The audience applauded the winner and there was good feeling all around.

There was only one hiccup in the show: the third couple of the three live sex acts. That contest was for the most artistic display of sexual intercourse. Think *Dancing with the Stars*, but the couple is naked and before the music ends there must be physical intimacy. The "betting" was based on the audience's vote tally for each couple; you had to get first-second-third in order, to be in the money. This guaranteed both audience and on-line participation.

The first couple did a tango to Brazilian music, with her stroking him at every contact. After a few minutes he entered her; they stayed erect and continued moving to the music, albeit at a much slower pace. When he was about to ejaculate they stopped and he held out his arms like Rio de Janeiro's giant Christ the Redeemer Statue. The whole act was very Brazilian, very effective.

The second couple danced to "Time of My Life," the final song of *Dirty Dancing*. They were the reincarnation of Patrick Swayze and Jennifer Grey from the movie, which many in the young audience had seen on TV. They were good! So good, I wondered what they were doing in this backwater Las Vegas cable show? But I forgot: buck naked just doesn't play well anywhere else. As he swung her around, she came closer and closer. He entered her and then the song climaxed, as did she (or simulated it).

Both couples were quite entertaining, and would be even more impressive with their clothes on. But then came the third couple, who began a dance to Pachelbel's Canon in D. It's not a dance piece, but they showed some nice steps to the ever popular Canon. This was Jerry and Juniper, the couple from Los Angeles, and I remembered they had mentioned something about a background in ballet. It showed, as they moved like professionals. Their plan was to consummate in bed, using balletic moves on the mattress. As they danced around naked, though, Jerry's problem became apparent. Whereas the other two guys had instant erections, he stayed limp. He and Juniper entered the bed, still struggling to show some artistry, but Juniper had to ad lib a bit, playing and fondling Jerry at every opportunity. Nothing worked.

I stood there like an idiot, not sure what to do. The two video guys didn't flinch and caught the non-action. The audience yelled out some suggestions.

"Get the Viagra."

"Cialis!"

"Hopewell, take over. She needs a man."

"Pull down your pants, Hopewell! Let her have it!"

"Hey, I'm available!"

Things start to get a little testy and the two bouncers, heretofore all but unseen on the side stairs, moved down toward the stage, ready to intervene if any audience members came forward. I half-expected Gabe or someone else to walk out from the wings and take over, but that didn't happen. When it became clear there would be no *consummation* for this act I moved stage-front.

"We seem to have a machinery malfunction," I announced. The audience tittered. "We will go to break, while our technicians work on the equipment." More tittering. My ad-libbing was not bad. Fortunately, the unseen person who controls what's shown on TV went right to a pre-taped commercial. The video guys shut down and I turned to talk with Jerry and Juniper.

"What's wrong?" I asked.

"He's had this problem occasionally. Nothing serious," said Juniper. "But it's not going to work tonight. After the break, tell them the equipment's been sent out for repairs."

"Shit, groused Jerry. I have no trouble in a real bed, with just us, but sometimes I just can't do it on command."

I was sympathetic. "I understand. I don't think I could ever do it before a live audience. No problem. Hey, go get dressed, I'll handle the audience." They left and stage hands removed the bed.

After the break I announced, "Welcome back, folks. Well, the equipment's been sent out for repairs, but won't be fixed in time for tonight's performance." This time laughter, with only one heckler.

"I'm still available!" he yelled.

"Yeah, but she's not," I replied. More laughter. "So we'll get on with our show."

I handled the situation well, more or less, and felt in synch with the audience. Yes, the whole experience was ego-satisfying, but I was also glad it was a one-time gig. I was out of character, in wig and fake mustache, ad-libbing before a live porn-show audience. That was certainly not what I trained for. I looked forward to returning to my own world, the hospital, and working without props.

But alas, the reward for good work is…more good work. Afterwards, Gabe and I met in his office to go over the show. I was feeling somewhat proud of myself and expected some praise. I got that, followed by a brick to my head.

"Good job tonight. You handled the Jerry and Juniper situation like a pro," Gabe said. "I held back, figuring you could take care of it."

"Thanks. They are nice people. I imagine this happens occasionally."

"Sometimes," he said.

"What do you do with the betting, since there's only two acts?"

"We'll figure it out. Another arm of Triple X works on that. Uh, Josh, I have some bad news."

"Oh?"

"Yes. Unfortunately, Brendan's not coming back."

"Not coming back? You mean on the show?"

"That's right. He's been arrested."

"Seriously? On what charge?"

"Prostitution. It's illegal in Vegas, in case you didn't know."

I sank in my chair. I really didn't want to know any details and just wanted to get the hell out of there. But I knew what was coming next.

"It's not going to be easy to find a new emcee. Brendan was a steal because he had a rap sheet. He wanted the work. A lot of guys, if they're any good, will rob you blind with demands."

Gabe rubbed his neck, as if he was trying to relieve tension. Or prepare me for a zinger.

"I think it's time to close the show," he said.

I looked hard at Gabe, annoyed at his method. Why couldn't he just say, 'Josh, you were wonderful out there, would you please consider staying on as emcee'? No, that wasn't his style. He put the dire consequence first. The question would come second. I asked it for him.

"So you want me to continue as emcee?"

"If you want. It's your investment."

"You mean, if we cancel, it's gone?"

"We've only done two shows. You're not getting your 100K back from those two. The real profit comes from the last three, when the cable audience is built up."

"What's the downside?"

"Downside?"

"Yes, of closing. Won't you lose money too, and what about your reputation?"

"Yes, of course, but this is my business. We have winners and losers. I'll survive. I really thought Brendan would last the six shows. My contract with the staff is for six shows, so I've got to pay them. As for you, you've got an honorable profession, I'm sure you'll recover."

I was surprised by the "honorable," as if to acknowledge his profession was not. But he was right about the recover part. Though I would be out most if not all of my 100K, it was money I could afford to lose. Doctors make bad investments all the time. I could chalk the whole thing up to 'experience', maybe even write a book about it. But no, I wouldn't, couldn't, let it go.

"So just four more shows?"

"Four more is what we're programmed for."

So there I was, minutes removed from stage success, now faced with the prospect of losing a ton of money versus returning to the stage and keeping my investment alive. The more I thought about it, under the circumstances, the decision seemed like a no-brainer.

"OK, I'll do it, but on one condition."

"I'm listening."

"You never divulge in public who I really am. You stick to my alias, no matter what."

"No problem."

———————◆———————

I got home around midnight. Barbara was up waiting for me.

"Josh, you were fantastic," she enthused. "It's the funniest thing I've seen in years."

"You watched it?"

"Irene called me right away. They were watching it. How did you end up on the show?"

"Josh, the anonymous porn host," I joked. "Madam, meet Mel Hopewell. Can I take your bet, my lady?"

"Yes," she said, with a pouty smile. "I'm betting on three climaxes tonight."

"I'll take that bet. If you go over, I win."

We laughed, then hugged. I remember feeling pretty good about myself that night.

———————◆———————

Gabe wasn't kidding about our emcee. A short article in the next day's paper headlined: "Prostitution ring busted, seven arrested." The names were listed, including "Brendan McKnight." Thankfully, there was no mention of *Consenting Adults Only*.

CHAPTER 20

—◆—

THAT I WAS IN LOVE with Barbara there was no doubt. Any doubts I had were about her past. I knew she came from a middle class family in Seattle, had gone to the University of Washington, majored in English, that kind of stuff. But what was her brief marriage like? Why did she choose a guy who was so unfaithful? And what was the secret she wouldn't reveal last month, when I 'pinky-swore' about my own past? And then there was the pole dancing. Sure, Irene was her best friend in Seattle, and Irene's pole dancing led Barbara to it. But was she inclined to exhibitionist behavior before moving to Las Vegas? Her work at the Trader John Saloon seemed so out of character for her background. But then, what do I know about pole dancers?

These were all nagging, almost subliminal questions, and would have stayed that way but for one seemingly minor situation in the ED.

I am not the jealous-boyfriend stereotype, suspicious of every guy in the room. It is inconceivable to me that a man would not know if his wife or live-in girlfriend was having an affair. Or a woman not know about her man. Yet you hear these things all the time, the spouse finding out months or years later. I mean, how could you not know? Surely there would be tell-tale signs in the bedroom, if not elsewhere. So I had no concerns about Barbara having physical intimacy with another man. My concern was about her *body language* around other men.

When I first met her back in October she turned me on, for sure, and that led to our dating, finding mutual attraction and then living together. Did I now expect Barbara to turn off her charms around other men? Well, yes, sort of, or at least not to flaunt them. But on more than one occasion I observed her too close to a male nurse, or bending over just a little too far so a guy could see her breasts, or smiling provocatively around a male physician.

The ED staff knew we were a couple, but I would not have been surprised if someone outside the ED asked her for a date. And then someone did: Dr. Smiley, a recently-divorced surgeon, handsome guy, in his late 30s. She worked with him in the ED on several occasions, when he came down to evaluate patients who might need general surgery. It may be, as I had observed around other men, that she was somewhat suggestive around Dr. Smiley: a blouse too open at the top, a smile that asked to be kissed, hips that got in the way in the small exam room. After finishing with his patient, Dr. Smiley asked if she would go for a cup of coffee later. She declined, said she was seeing someone. He replied that she should "let me know if you're ever available. I think you're a great nurse and I would love to sit and chat."

And I knew what else he would love to do, of course. Anyway, I found out about this from a nurse's aide who overheard the innocent conversation, a woman named Cecelia. In her early 30s, from Arkansas, Cecelia was not the most educated of our staff, but she was efficient and competent. She was herself married, and apparently wise to the ways of both men and women. Anyway, Cecelia came up to me the next day, and in a friendly Arkansas twang said, "Doc, you better watch that honey of yours, Guys 'll be askin' her out."

"Oh?"

"Yeah, Doc Smiley did yesterday." She recounted the event, including Barbara's response, then said: "I knows you two is a couple, so I'm just trying to patch the tire before it springs a leak." She was not being gossipy or vengeful or anything negative, just Arkansas-honest. Her comment was incisive.

I had to bring this up with Barbara. But bring up what exactly? That a guy asked her out and she said no? Maybe I *am* the jealous-boyfriend stereotype. If I was Barbara, I would reply, "and don't you fantasize screwing every beautiful woman you see? Give me a break." Mostly true, if she said that. So what was I going to complain about? I didn't know, but just had to get it off my chest. I waited until we got into bed.

"I heard Dr. Smiley asked you out."

"Oh, Cecelia told you? Girl has a big mouth. Did she tell you I said yes, that we went for coffee and then made sweet, passionate love?"

"Barbara, don't taunt me like that."

"Well, I can't help it if men find me attractive. You did."

"I know, but now that I have you, I do think you could be, I don't know, less provocative."

"What do you mean?"

"I mean, you do turn men on. You may not be fully aware, but sometimes with your body language, that's all. It's provocative. Maybe you still have pole dancing in you."

"I wouldn't talk. Who's the host of a porn show? Who gets a kick out of people going to the bathroom to lose weight?"

"OK, OK, let's not argue, I said. It's just a concern I have."

I lit a fuse and was not prepared for the coming explosion.

"And while we're at it," she said, "what about that crazy bitch who keeps trying to mess us up? I haven't been complaining about your Judy. What do you do to turn her on, that she keeps coming back? You think I don't know about the letter she sent?"

"What?"

"You got a letter from Judy."

"How do you know that?"

"She told me."

"Who told you?" I could only think of Dr. Sobel.

"Judy sent me a note. I threw it away. Wanted to see if you would tell me yourself. You never did, and so I assumed it was a crazy letter and you ignored it. I knew what she wanted, to come between us, and I wasn't going to let it happen."

"What'd the note say?"

"Something about a letter she sent you that would finish us off, and she was sorry, dear, but that's the way the cookie crumbles. Really crazy, just like she is. But now you bring up my behavior around men. What do you do that keeps attracting Judy? Or am I not allowed to ask?"

I had no answer for her.

"I mean, for God's sake, Josh, I work with Dr. Smiley. So he likes me and asks me out. I don't hesitate to say no, and that's that. But Judy, she keeps coming back and back and back. And not in a way friendly to yours truly. How do you explain that?"

"OK, I'm sorry I brought it up. Forget it."

"I can't forget it, Josh. You keep probing me, looking for a deep dark secret."

"I'm sorry, forget it."

"I can't forget it. OK, you want to know my fucking secret?"

"Whatever you want Barbara."

"OK. I was molested. Sexually abused. By my uncle, when I was eight. And nine. Over eighteen months. He fondled me, played with me, and then he fucked me ten, fifteen times. I lost count. Said it was an uncle's love. Said if I told my father, his brother, he'd hurt me, too. Gave me toys, dolls, acted so loving. And he did it to me for a year and a half. A little girl! My parents never knew. I wanted to tell them, to get away from him, but I was a child. I was afraid they would blame me, and things would just get worse. So I suffered in silence. How's that for some scars on your life?"

For a moment I didn't know what to say. A question seemed appropriate.

"What happened that it stopped?"

"Providence happened. He was killed in car crash. My father mourned. I didn't. I was so relieved. I had to hide my happiness."

"Where was your sister when all this took place?"

"She was only four. My uncle babysat for us when Mom and Dad went out. He didn't mess with her. Figured she didn't have the maturity to stay quiet. But with me it was all cuddly love. Until it wasn't."

"Did you get therapy, any help?"

"For what? I got puberty is what I got, then a real sexual desire, and I put the past behind me. Then I found a guy in college who I loved, in part because he was so loving in bed, so kind and gentle. And you know what happened there. Then I find you. And you complain about my flirting with other men, even though I am not trying to, and have no intention to?"

I could feel her getting angry. I fumbled with what to say next, to defuse her anger and at the same time offer some help. I failed. Miserably.

"Barbara, I'm sorry. I'm sorry for your past, and that you waited so long to tell me. I'm sorry I questioned your intentions. I am concerned for you, that's all. There's something there, I don't know. Your uncle, your ex-husband, the pole dancing, what happened in the limousine. I'm just concerned, that's all. I'm being honest. Would you consider seeing a therapist?"

"Would you?" Her retort was quick, almost instinctive.

"For what?"

"For what? For WHAT? You think this little rift is just about Barbara's past? What about *your* past that makes you go for Judy, and porno, and bathroom elimination contests?"

"I didn't have any childhood trauma, thankfully. And I dumped Judy because I knew she wasn't for me, and never intended to marry her. And the porn show, that was just a foolish investment, a one-time thing. I don't need to see a therapist. But you..."

"Really? So it's just me? IS THAT WHAT YOU'RE FUCKING SAYING? IT'S JUST ME? I'M OUT OF HERE!"

She got up to leave, wearing only a nightgown. The bedroom night-light outlined her figure. She stood on the side of the bed, looked down at me. "JOSH, YOU'RE A FUCKING ASS HOLE!" She made for the door.

I was about to lose her, and this time I knew she would not come back. I ran to the bedroom door and blocked it just as she reached for the doorknob.

"Barbara listen, please." She pounded my chest with both arms and started crying.

"Let me go! Let me go!"

"No please, listen, please." She ran to the far corner of the room and fell to the ground, curled up, crying. I put my arms around her.

"Barbara, Barbara. It's OK, I'm here."

"No you're not here, Josh. You're really not here. You have no understanding. None at all."

I have no understanding? Is that what she said? And then it hit me. I really didn't have a clue. And our relationship was about to break apart. Not because either of us was unfaithful, but because I had no understanding. Now I had to make a choice, one that couldn't be put off if I wanted to keep her: either attempt repairs or let it go.

We stayed on the floor a good ten minutes, she in the fetal position, me holding her, no words spoken. When she stopped crying, I said, "Barbara, if you'll come back to bed, and not leave me, I promise I will set up appointments for both of us, for couple's therapy. I don't want us to break apart. I will do whatever it takes, I promise."

Slowly, she rose from the floor and let me assist her back to bed. I held her in bed until we both fell asleep. When I awoke in the morning she was still there.

———————

The next day I called Dr. Sobel.

"Rose, I just have a quick question, if you have a minute."

"Sure, Josh."

"This situation with Judy I talked to you about is affecting my relationship with Barbara, the woman I'm living with. I think we both need to talk to a really good therapist about our issues. Can you recommend someone?"

"Sure, I understand. You know I don't do therapy, so I'm going to give you two names, in order of preference. They're both women, is that alright?"

"Sure. I think a woman will understand these issues better than a man."

She gave me the names. I knew neither therapist. I called the first one, a Ph.D. named Molly Siegel, left a voice message on her answering machine that mentioned Dr. Sobel and my desire for couple's therapy. She called back later that day.

"Dr. Luvkin, just explain briefly what the issue is, why you think you need couple's therapy. I want to make sure I can help."

"Sure. I'm in love with a nurse I work with, Barbara. We live together, will probably get married. I'm being stalked by an ex-girlfriend who Barbara perceives as a threat to our relationship. Actually, I feel that way too. At the same time I'm concerned that Barbara is turning on other men in a way that she is unaware of. And to be honest, she is concerned that I am somehow encouraging my ex-girlfriend, but that's definitely not the case. I am currently hosting a cable porn show and she brings that up to suggest there's maybe something wrong with me. All this stuff is getting so intertwined it's creating a lot of tension in our relationship. A lot."

"Sounds like a novel. All this is really happening, now?"

"I'm afraid so." Was Dr. Siegel overwhelmed by my brief description? Maybe I should have just said 'we're having some disagreement' and not crammed everything in.

"Well," she said, "from your brief description, all this may take some time to work through. Typically several sessions, maybe more. Are you both committed to that?"

"I think we have to be," I said. "We're ready."

I got an appointment for later in the week.

CHAPTER 21

―――――

DR. SIEGEL IS ABOUT THE same age as Dr. Sobel, mid 50s, with a thriving practice in downtown Vegas, close to my attorney's office. Our first appointment was for ninety minutes, with the promise of subsequent hours depending on how things went.

Unlike many of my medical school classmates and residency colleagues, I never sought psychological counseling. Never had the need to. Call it a healthy ego or whatever, that's the way I felt. Even now, I still figured this was not about me so much, but more about Barbara and how her makeup affected our relationship. This thought made it easy to rationalize what my well-defended self was doing in a psychologist's office.

Dr. Siegel's office was like a large home study, nicely carpeted, with book cases, couch, chairs and desk, all in good taste. She arranged three comfortable chairs for the sessions, so that Barbara and I sat facing her. She did not use a computer but a just a yellow pad to write occasional notes as we talked.

"The way I would like to do this," she said at the beginning, "is to work with you together, never separately. That way there are no secrets in therapy, no wondering what the other person told me. Sometimes the husband or wife will try to contact me privately, to explain something they didn't want their spouse to hear. I don't allow that, it's never helpful to me. So is this acceptable to both of you? I understand you're not married but the situation is really the same."

We both nodded yes.

She then began to take our histories, starting with me. The first session was somewhat painful. She probed gently, but my answers often seemed to give her pause. She wanted to know my reasons for delaying medical school, about my relationship with Mom and Dad. I told her briefly about Yellowstone, Wendy and India.

"That's when you decided to go to medical school, in Delhi? Tell me about that." I had never gotten around to telling Barbara the story, because it seemed so un-Josh-like she might not believe it.

"It's trivial in the scheme of things, just something that happened to me, and helped make my decision."

"Well, I want to hear it. That's why we're here."

"After I broke up with Wendy, I toured the country, first with a buddy, and then alone. When I was in Delhi, this was now about five months after I arrived, I was staying alone in a hotel. There was a monument I still wanted to see, one of the World Heritage sites called Qutb Minar. I was into monuments then."

I paused, waiting for her to say, "OK, that's enough, let's move on." Of course she didn't say that. She didn't say anything.

"From my hotel I figured public transportation would take half a day for the ten-mile trip. For twenty dollars prepaid I was able to hire a car and driver for the afternoon. The monument was certainly worth seeing, and I stayed well over an hour. We started the drive back about an hour before sundown. On the way back we got stuck in traffic. Have you been to India?" I asked.

"No," she said, "but I hear it's crowded."

"Yeah, well, traffic can stop dead almost anytime, anywhere, from a cow, an accident, a demonstration, a large pot hole. Anyway, it was now near sundown and I was in the back seat. My driver was a man named Rangu, probably in his late 30s. We had made desultory conversation to this point, but he became more conversant when we stopped moving.

"We got to talking, waiting for things to clear on the road. Nice guy, but clearly annoyed with the stop and go traffic. This was a busy two-lane road, and on most such roads in Delhi people also walk on the sides, carrying laundry, food, furniture or just themselves. At this point the walkers were at an advantage. Cars were not moving, for no apparent reason we could see. Just then tapping began at my window."

I realized I was not so much relating an event but telling a story. I was building suspense, sort of like the stories I've told to my niece and nephew. Is this what she wanted? Or should I just say I gave a begging women some rupees and be done with it? I decided the story was better – to tell the event the way I experienced it. If Dr. Siegel or Barbara were bored they didn't show it. My thought paused the story and Dr. Siegel asked, "Who was tapping?"

"Oh, it was a young Indian woman dressed in colorful rags, holding an infant. Nothing new, of course, they are all over the streets. I even heard "begging managers" rent out babies in the morning, to increase the begging proceeds. At night the babies are returned, to be sent out again the next day.

"Anyway, my driver right away said, "Don't respond Mr. Loofkin." I pronounced my name just the way he did, for verisimilitude. "Will just bring more out," he said.

"But the woman kept tapping. Having a driver, and with my appearance, she knew I was a foreigner and therefore a rich target. I couldn't help but look at her. She had that look, what I would describe as National Geographic poor. You know the images: face gaunt, eyes wide open, pleading."

"Sounds like an uncomfortable situation," said Dr. Siegel.

"Well, for me it was. My driver Rangu saw me glance at the woman. Right away he said, "Don't look! No eye contact. Brings others." He was pretty emphatic. Then he started honking his horn, clearly annoyed with the stalled traffic."

"So I obeyed and stared straight ahead, but feeling more uncomfortable by the minute. However my brief look had encouraged the woman. The baby started crying, as if on cue. I wondered if she had pinched the child. And the woman did not stop tapping the window. I remember to this day. Tap, tap, tap. And we were stuck, no movement. So I started to roll down the window. I figured maybe a dollar would satisfy her and make her go away. Well you can imagine my driver when I did that. He implored me, "Don't roll down the window, Mr. Loofkin, please." It was a hellish moment. Rangu was honking his horn, the baby was crying, the woman was tapping the half open window. Tap, tap, tap, tap, tap."

"You're painting a vivid picture," said Dr. Siegel. "Please continue."

"So I looked straight at the woman. Her eyes implored for a handout. Then she held the baby out a few inches with one arm, and with the other arm put two fingers to her lips. I knew what she meant: *My baby is hungry.*"

"I lost it, I have to admit. At that time I thought of my own niece at home, only a year old when I left. You know, happy, healthy in America, and this baby hungry in India. I simply could not bear it any longer, so I opened the door. Right away, Rangu said "Where are you going?"

As I got out of the car I said, "Leave me here, Rangu. I'll walk back to the hotel." Then I shut the door. As luck would have it, just then traffic began to move and the car behind honked. Rangu was not moving quickly enough, since he had been distracted by my hasty exit. He caught up with the traffic, but looked back to see if I would run up and get in the car. I waved him to go on."

"So you're there alone," asked Dr. Siegel, "on the side of this busy street, with a woman and baby asking for a handout?"

"Yeah, and I forgot Rangu's car was air-conditioned. Outside was hot, muggy and smelly. A mixture of dirt, perhaps, with a hint body odor and excrement. I remember feeling slightly disoriented. Suddenly there were people all around me, ordinary Indians, which is to say poor. Several approached, but first the woman with child. Her eyes fixed on mine. There was no shame or anything, only want. So I pulled out some bills, gave her an American dollar and fifty rupees. Then everyone else stretched out hands. I know I invited this, indeed expected it. Certainly I had been warned."

"What'd you do?"

"I began distributing all the money I had, about twenty-five American dollars, plus another ten in rupees. I filled each outstretched hand with a little bit of paper money and was done in five minutes. The only thing left when I was done were my passport and credit card, in an inside pants pocket. But even so, more beggars came, and implored me in their native tongue. I heard no English at all. I showed them my pockets were empty. No more, I said, over and over. So gradually they walked away, to look for handouts elsewhere.

"Then the tapping woman came up to me. She no longer had the baby. I guess it had served its purpose. Who knows? Maybe with another beggar. Anyway, she grabbed my hand and kissed it. Then she bowed and walked away."

"What then?"

"So by now it was dark. I was sweaty, out in the open. I had about two miles back to the hotel. Fortunately the hotel was on the same road, so I knew where to go. I walked the distance, unmolested. To this day I don't know why I acted so impulsively, against all advice, but was glad I did. Something changed at that moment in India. That's when I made my decision. The next day I called my parents and told them I was coming home, that I wanted to go to medical school."

"Interesting story," said Dr. Siegel. "Thanks for sharing it. But what in this event changed your mind?"

"I just felt good helping this woman. I liked the feeling. I was probably half-way there already, what with my family background and my parents' stated wishes. But this was the catalyst. But I must tell you, before my encounter with the woman I had not committed to any career path. Medical school was just one of many options. On my walk back to the hotel it became my only option. Happened fast."

I was glad I had told the event in storybook fashion. Clearly Dr. Siegel was impressed. I figured Barbara was, too, though she didn't speak up during the telling. But kudos weren't forthcoming, and her next question surprised me a bit. "Do you think you're different now, that being financially successful has somehow changed you?"

"No," I answered, perhaps a little too quickly. I saw an eyebrow rise up but she asked no more about that. Of course her question nagged at me. If a friend had asked that question I would have retorted with a defensive "What do you mean?" but my therapist was not my friend. She was just probing, getting a good sense of my situation. I rationalized that her ultimate goal was not so much to make me a better person as to make us a healthier couple, and let it go.

She moved on to my relationship with Judy. After I explained the situation and what happened when Barbara and Judy first met, she brought Barbara into the conversation.

"Barbara, what did you think then?"

"I didn't know what to think, only that I had to get out of there. If he was really married that was going to be the end of our relationship, of that I was certain. I felt a little better when he called the next day, but was not ready to reconcile. I was married once, to a loser, and wasn't going to fall for another one."

So far nothing had been mentioned about her childhood. To get into her early years Dr. Siegel's question was rather direct, I thought. "Barbara, how old were you when you first had sexual intercourse?"

Barbara looked at me, perhaps wondering if I said something on the initial phone call. I had not, of course.

"Eight. Eight years old."

Dr. Siegel did not show any surprise. "Tell me about it," she said.

Barbara's story was horrific. Dr. Siegel asked her to recount the sexual abuse in more detail than I wanted to hear. I squirmed, wanted to go kill her uncle but he was already dead. After just one such account Dr. Siegel backed off, and concentrated more on Barbara's failed marriage, the pole dancing, and her relationship with Irene.

"Were you and Irene ever lovers?"

Another direct question that caught me by surprise. Frankly, I never considered the possibility.

"No, never. Never even thought about it." I tried to show no emotion but inwardly felt very relieved. Bi-sexuality -- even history thereof -- was not a trait I wanted in my mate for life.

"Tell me about the pole dancing."

Barbara was of course much more open with Dr. Siegel than she had been with me on our first date. For some reason, when Barbara described the sordidness of Trader Johns, Dr. Siegel nodded in affirmation. Had our therapist been there? Did she ever pole dance? I so wanted to ask.

Then she got into the rape.

"After that incident, what made you want to continue at Trader Johns?"

"Really, the money," Barbara said. "The assault was outside the club. What happened was in part my own fault."

"How so?"

Barbara started to cry. Dr. Siegel leaned over and handed her some tissues.

"Do you two want to take a little break? We can resume in a few minutes."

"No, no, it's OK," said Barbara. "I'm fine. I meant the pregnancy. That was in part my fault."

"You became pregnant?"

I interjected. "Dr. Siegel, she became pregnant from the assault, and had an abortion at eight weeks. I think that's why Barbara's so upset now. It's weighed heavily on her ever since."

Barbara nodded in affirmation but did not elaborate.

"I understand," Dr. Siegel replied.

I thought her reply was gratuitous and my impulse was to blurt out 'NO, you don't understand. Did you ever get raped and have an abortion'? I'm glad I checked my impulse, especially as I reflect on what Dr. Siegel really meant: the explanation for Barbara's emotion was rational, made sense.

Dr. Siegel than asked Barbara about any other affairs. There was one, in nursing school, but she used the pill and broke up with the guy after six months. Barbara had mentioned this before our sessions began and I never probed for details.

Dr. Siegel than returned to me, and I brought her up to speed on the recent events with the porn show. She was not judgmental, just more probing.

"Have you always been interested in porn?"

"Excuse me?"

"I mean, did you have an interest in pornography before this business venture. Are you into porn? TV? Internet? Magazines. I'm not being judgmental. Just trying to get a better feel for your background."

"I'm not into porn at all. I don't watch it, download it, or go to peep shows. This was a kinky business deal, that's all."

"Did you ever consider just saying no?"

"All the time."

"And why didn't you?"

"I don't know. Sounded like a way to make a lot of money in some area totally different from medicine. Some doctors invest in restaurants, I invested in a cable show. Both are pretty far removed from the practice of medicine."

"And you like this side job?"

"I don't dislike it. I find it intriguing. I certainly did not intend to be a porn show host. This just sort of happened to me, as I explained. So I'm going to finish with it, then I'll be done."

"I still find it unusual that someone with your background would undertake such an adventure. Were you exposed to pornography growing up?"

Now I was getting defensive. I remembered Gabe's comment: *Why is sex pornography, but murder and mayhem are not?*

"Do you mean pictures of the sex act?"

"Actually, I mean anything your family or friends would have considered pornographic. I'm not here to pass any judgment, just trying to figure out what's motivating you two."

I hesitated. Barbara looked at me.

"When I was a kid, eleven or twelve. I was looking for some missing comic books. I thought my mom had put them somewhere, maybe hid them from me. She kept telling me I was too old to read that junk. Couldn't find them, so I went through the closet in their bedroom when they weren't home. And I found a box on my father's side, under some shirts."

"Your comic books?"

"Hardly. My father's porn stash."

"Very interesting," Dr. Siegel said, a comment I thought both reflexive and a touch unprofessional.

"Do you mind telling me about it?" she asked.

Barbara fidgeted, then looked at me raised eyebrows, which was surprising. Compared to her childhood, this bit of history was rather mundane.

"Photographs and videos," I said. "VHS at the time. Mom and Dad, I couldn't believe it. But there was more. Professional, mail-order videos. Certainly people I didn't know."

By way of further explanation, I looked at Barbara and said, "Sort of like the video Carl and Irene made."

"Carl is?" asked Dr. Siegel.

"Irene's husband. They made a porn video for Triple X. Carl's the one who connected me to the Triple X producer."

"I see. So your friend made a porn video. Were either of you in it?"

"Oh, no, no," I said. "Just Carl and his wife. But it was done professionally, for sale by the cable channel."

"But you've both seen it?"

"Yes," I said. Barbara nodded yes as well.

Dr. Siegel scribbled some notes.

"Getting back to the videos you found as a child, did they show your father with another woman, not your mother?"

"No, thank God."

"But you watched the videos?"

"Yes, couldn't help it. But not the amateur ones with my parents. After a few minutes of that I didn't want to see any more, and rewound it.

But the others, I watched when they weren't home, then put them back just the way I found them."

"How many would you say?"

"I don't know, maybe ten."

"More than once?"

"Some of them."

"Did you ever confront your parents?"

"No, never. Way too embarrassed."

"So they never knew you went rummaging?"

"Not as far as I know."

"And as a teenager?"

"What?"

"Seek out porn as a teenager?"

"Well, the usual girlie magazines, that kind of stuff. The boys all did that. But we never went to sex shops or anything."

"College?"

"Well, at parties, there was sometimes a back room with movies that might be considered pornography. Nothing special. In truth, by that time I was fully able to find real girls and I had no interest in porn. I know this may sound strange, but porn has never been my thing."

"But your father, you said he was into it when you were a kid."

"Yes, judging by his stash. And, I guess, with my mother's approval. I mean, she was in some of the videos."

"Made in their bedroom? Could you tell?"

"Oh, yes, right in our home."

"I see."

What did she see? That I had a genetic predisposition to pornography? A familial bent? That both Barbara and I had these little skeletons in our closets? At least in my case, it wasn't such a big deal. My guess is that she saw a disturbing pattern of experiences and behavior. There was no disputing the facts:

Barbara: childhood rape by uncle; early marriage to a philanderer; best friend a pole dancer; she takes up pole dancing; raped in limousine;

on first date with doctor, willingly goes to excretion contest and then goes to bed with him.

Josh: childhood fascination with father's porn stash; could move anywhere after medical training but chose Sin City; sexual relationship with a borderline woman; fascinated with Biggest Loser contests; attracted to pole dancer; jumps at chance to invest in porn show; does not turn down opportunity to host the show.

I could guess what Dr. Siegel was probably thinking about us. *Unhealthy attraction to pornography. Each has formed relationships with unstable partners. How will they ever stay faithful to one another?* I could not argue with that line of thinking, given the combined histories as they unfolded. But I was not pessimistic. The damning list of past events did not, in my mind, predict anything. I felt my relationship with Barbara was special, what most people would identify as simply being in love.

Once past the history-taking sessions I felt more comfortable. The act of talking to Dr. Siegel, and making sure there were no secrets, was helpful. We learned a few things about each other not known before, and as result became more trusting; the "Fucking Asshole" scene receded in memory.

There was no score card to these sessions, no summary of blame, but there was, I have to admit, some not-too-favorable analysis that Dr. Siegel shared with us. Nothing surprising. For Barbara: a tendency to exhibitionism, a heightened desire to be loved physically and emotionally that unconsciously caused her to flirt, and an unconscious need to wash away past sins. For me: a tendency to objectify women, a somewhat shallow approach to emotional involvement, an unconscious desire for pornographic display, and not enough superego to say no when I should.

These assessments frankly didn't mean much to me. They were a psychologist's description of character flaws, for which there is no antidote. Which is not to be critical of her analysis, not at all. I had never thought about my situation in terms of character flaws, and now I did. But it had to be put in perspective. Don't we all have flaws? So what?

If we can learn to accept our makeup, stay happy and healthy and not harm others, so what?

In truth I was accepting and appreciative of her assessments. Dr. Siegel was, in the end, extremely helpful. What we got out of the sessions was a deeper appreciation of our pasts, and knowledge that if we loved *and trusted* each other, our relationship could be solid.

———◆———

I did two more shows as Mel Hopewell, all under the radar. By now *Consenting Adults Only* had generated some word-of-mouth publicity, and Gabe only had to distribute a thousand flyers to fill the auditorium. I got through the next two shows with wig and moustache, and no one to my knowledge recognized me. My inner circle thought it was a hoot. I thought, maybe I have some talent for TV hosting. *This could be a side career.*

What happened next was, I suppose, inevitable. A middle-aged man came to the ED with an acute ankle sprain and tibial bone contusion, after falling off a ladder at home. X-rays showed no fracture, but he was in a lot of pain from the fall. All he needed was a brace, pair of crutches and prescription for some pain medication. As I was prepared to discharge him, he asked,

"Say, Dr. Luvkin, you look just like the guy my wife and I saw at a live TV show last week. *Consenting Adults Only.* You sound like him, too. Great show!"

So I was recognized. Do I lie and say *no, you're mistaken, sir, here's your prescription see you later.* Or, *no, he's my twin brother, but we sure do look alike, don't we?*

I liked the second ploy, especially if delivered semi-sarcastically, leaving the possibility that I am joking.

"Nah, must be my twin brother," I replied.

"Yeah, then why does he have a different name, Doc?"

Caught! I smiled and winked at him. *Shut up, already.*

"I get it, Doc. Great job."

I shooed him out the door, but knew there would be more of "Hey, aren't you..." soon. I am sure Dr. Oz cannot operate on a patient without some banter back and forth about his TV gig. Of course his gig is all about helping people. Mine is about titillating them. Porn, if you want to be technical about it.

I could put up with the occasional patient recognition, even knowledge among staff that "Dr. Luvkin has another job, hosting a porn show." I figured most would never watch it, and in any case, if I did my medical job reasonably well it really shouldn't matter. But I was not prepared for widespread publicity. For some reason, I thought the show would be hidden from the general TV-watching public, far below the news media radar. Boy, was I wrong. After just four shows had aired the following review appeared in the *Las Vegas Sun*, in the widely read weekly column "The Tube" by Bill Pierce. Pierce covers TV and local media. The headline said it all.

The Tube
By Bill Pierce

Disgusting

OK, let's get this out of the way now. Anything goes in Vegas, and to complain about defecation contests and live sex acts must make me seem like a first-class prude. But the new show on local cable channel XXX-Las Vegas is, in a word, disgusting. Called *Consenting Adults Only*, part of the show is taken up with contests that include weight loss after a single bathroom visit (aka The Biggest Loser, but this one is not about dieting) and which contestant couple has the most artistic fornication. Then there is sex in unusual situations (sky diving, scuba diving, bicycling) or "10 positions you didn't know existed." Oh, and the ads: demonstrations of new masturbatory toys is a biggie. All of this is before a live audience, though a part of each show is on video. The audience seems to buy into it, since the free studio tickets are apparently hard to come by.

There is some good news. The show has no bestiality, no child porn (which of course would be completely illegal) and no sado-masochism. In fact, that's the business model. Co-producer Gabe Stein says the show will never air anything that isn't between consenting adults or that is perceived to inflict physical or emotional harm. So only warm, cuddly stuff. What about homosexuality? Stein: "XXX-Vegas has other shows for homosexuals that are clearly labeled as such. Our target audience is heterosexual, so we don't plan on showing homosexual activity."

And the other co-producer? None other than the new host of the show, Mel Hopewell. As in, Hope all is Well. Nah. That's not his real name. He is Dr. Joshua Luvkin, a doctor, for God sakes. When not co-producing and hosting *Consenting Adults Only* he works shifts at the Memorial Hospital Emergency Department. I was able to reach him by phone. He seemed embarrassed by the gig, and our conversation was short. He did say: "Dr. Oz was a heart surgeon before entering television, so there is precedent." Of course, Dr. Oz gives out useful information. This show gives out bulls- - -. Oh, wait, I'm wrong: it's the human variety.

OK, you can call me a prude. But if this stuff interests you, then we have a little disagreement. I found much of the show repulsive. But hey, this is what makes Vegas, Vegas. Let's just hope this crap "stays here" and doesn't migrate to normal America.

I do remember the phone call. Pierce had caught me off guard. Why is a reporter from the newspaper calling me? About the show? Oh, yes, I told him, I was the host. How did he find out?

"A reporter has his sources, Doc. Then I see you are listed as co-producer, along with Mr. Stein?"

"Really? How'd you find that out?"

"Hey doc, every TV show has to have an FCC license, listing the pro-ducers. You're right there. I just googled it."

"Oh," was all I could manage. I so wanted to make my host role rel-evant to medicine, I did mumble something about Dr. Oz. He shot back with, "do you think peddling crap is the same as offering good advice on daytime TV?" It was obvious he was not a fan. I felt blind-sided, and said I had to go take care of patients. Yes the conversation was brief, but obviously not brief enough.

Although negative, the review left me with a mixed reaction. The oft-repeated mantra, "Even bad publicity is good publicity" certainly was in the show's favor. There are people out there who find this stuff enter-taining, who might read Pearson's review and think 'Wow!

This is just what I'm looking for'.

On the other hand, the review probably ended forever my medical career, at least on this planet. Who would want an ED doctor who wal-lows in porn? I envisioned a scene in the ED:

"Dr. Luvkin will see you now."

"Dr. Luvkin? From Triple X-Las Vegas? I don't think so. I'm taking my heart attack out of here unless you find me a new doctor."

And if I ever applied for another job as emergency medicine physician:

"I see you've applied for a position here in Nome General, Alaska's northern-most hospital. I'm sorry, Dr. Luvkin, but that position just filled this morning."

At least those were my thoughts at the time.

CHAPTER 22

———

I WAITED FOR THE INEVITABLE call. It came from Dr. John Billington's secretary. "Dr. Billington would like to set up a meeting with you as soon as possible." I knew what it was about, so didn't even ask.

We met the next day in his office. He also invited the hospital's general counsel, Margaret Rachaelson. She's in her mid-40s, with a tough-as-nails reputation. I had met her once, at a meeting a year ago, and was sure she didn't know me from Adam. We said hello, shook hands and I took my seat.

"Josh, I suppose you know what this is about," John began. "Before we make any comments, could you just give us some background on this affair?" He held up Pierce's newspaper review. "What's it all about?"

"Excuse me, John," said Mrs. Rachaelson. "Josh, do you mind if I tape this meeting? I need your permission to do so."

"No, that's fine." I appreciated the warning, so I wouldn't say anything stupid or defamatory. She pulled out her smart phone and entered a few clicks.

"We're ready," she said.

I recounted the full story, explained how the cable show was just an investment and how I had zero intention of ever going on camera. I explained it was a desperation ploy to protect my investment. I was contrite for the result, but not apologetic for the attempt.

"If you think about it, doctors invest in Broadway shows," I said. "Why can't a doctor invest in a porn show? Realistically, had I not done the emcee job no one would even know or care."

"Well," interjected Mrs. Rachaelson, "I agree, but here's the issue. You of course have every right to your business interests, unless they directly conflict with the hospital's business. Under the terms of your contract, for example, you could not set up your own Urgent Care center while working here. That's fairly straightforward. Also, your contract does allow the hospital to take action against a physician "for cause." This means, if you are medically incompetent, or you become what's known as a disruptive physician, we can initiate proceedings that might result in dismissal. "For cause," of course, would also include anything blatantly illegal, such as a felony."

She was poised and professional. This meeting was probably just a line item in her busy schedule: 'meet with MD re: porn show'. She sat erect in a straight-back chair, regal-like, and was dressed in a smart business suit. I also couldn't help noting the rock on her finger, the size of a golf ball. My mind wandered. *She probably makes more than I do.*

"None of these items pertain, here," she continued. "You've committed no crime, and from what I understand your patient care is exemplary." I nodded my head in agreement.

"Then we come to the gray area of bad publicity, which is your situation. The reality is you've indirectly – and believe me, we understand this was unintentional – you've indirectly sullied the hospital's reputation, which is really why we're here. So right now, to be honest, I don't see anything illegal. I explained this assessment to Dr. Billington coming in. We just want to discuss this with you. Call it damage control."

"Thanks for the explanation," I said, trying my hardest to be sincere and not sound sarcastic.

"First of all," said John, "I want to be clear we're not going to try to boot you off the staff or short-circuit your career here at Memorial.

We're not Neanderthals. On the other hand, frankly Josh, we don't want any more bad publicity. How do *you* think we should handle this?"

"I'm just curious," I replied. "Has there been any direct fallout so far?"

Billington looked at Rachaelson. "Frankly yes, he said. I've already been called by two local papers for a statement. We've put them off."

I swallowed hard. *Damn. This really is a big deal.* "I appreciate your concerns, I really do. I am in this investment thing to $100,000. And if you think the hospital is besmirched, imagine my own chagrin. I'm just glad I don't have any family in town."

Mrs. Diamond Ring twisted the rock on her finger ever so slightly. Body English to tell me she does have a family.

"I don't see any choice here," I continued. "My medical career is obviously more important than any stupid cable show. The only thing left for me to do is quit the show. By contract there are only two more shows planned, but I won't be hosting them. However, there is nothing I can do about re-runs, which I understand are a big part of their business plan."

"Yes, we figured as much, and there is probably nothing we can do about it legally," said John. "But if you're willing to quit, I think we can craft a statement for the papers, and then this will blow over. The one advantage is being in Las Vegas, this kind of stuff never lingers."

"Well, it's not so simple, John," said Rachaelson. "My office has done some investigation of this Triple X cable company. Turns out they are under investigation by both the IRS and the Nevada Gaming Commission."

"Oh, I didn't know that, Margaret. Did you Josh?"

"Me? No, not at all."

"So what does this mean, Margaret?" he asked. John was CEO but for the moment it appeared Margaret Rachaelson was in charge.

"On the surface, not much. The investigation has to do with an off-shore betting affiliate connected in some way with Triple X. The affiliate handles betting for the cable channel. There's an issue of whether it complies with United States and Nevada gambling regulations, and also whether Triple X has paid all taxes due on wagers collected. They've received letters from the state and the IRS, and formal complaints have been filed. This usually leads to a hearing and there's always the possibility of a criminal indictment."

"I assure you," I said, rather defensively, "I had nothing to do with the betting. All this is new to me."

"But you do have a contract with Triple X?"

"Well, yes."

"Do you remember if your percentage of profit mentioned anything about betting?"

In fact it did. I had gone over the issue with Gabe and then with Dworkin. "Yes, but I wasn't involved in setting up any betting arrangements."

"I'm sure not," she said. "The issue is, if you quit the emcee job today, you're still a party to the contract. If the papers want to pursue this, you're still a principal of the show, you're still connected. And if there is a hint of illegality or tax evasion, it's just more bad publicity. My point, John, is that Dr. Luvkin has to quit the show in person *and* contractually. Our statement has to state he has nothing more to do with the cable company in any way, shape or manner."

This was some smart attorney. She had me by the balls.

"Do you get what she's saying, Josh?"

"I think so. How exactly do I quit contractually?"

"Obviously, no one at the hospital can represent you," she replied. "Do you have a contract attorney?"

"Yes, Harold Dworkin. His office is downtown."

She gave no reaction to the name, which evidently meant nothing to her.

"Talk to him, today if possible. We need you to get out of the contract, then we can answer the papers."

I saw my investment evaporate. No contract, no money. I remember Harold's comment about Gabe: *If the contract lets him get away with something, he'll more than likely try it.* Without any contract, I imagined Gabe could get away with a lot more: everything, in fact.

"That's 100,000 dollars," I protested.

"I don't know how your contract reads, but if you've already done four shows, you should be able to get something back, if not all of it. Talk to your attorney. Let me be clear. I represent the hospital. My advice is based only on what I perceive is best for the hospital. You remain free to do as you choose, and I am not, strictly speaking, giving you legal advice. If you don't cancel your contract with Triple X, we can still issue a statement, saying you're no longer with the show. I just don't want some enterprising reporter digging up dirt and writing how Memorial's ED physician is still a principal with one of Triple X's shows. So it's up to you, and how Dr. Billington wants to handle the situation."

"Thanks, Margaret," said the CEO. "You've been most helpful, as always. Anything else you think we need to know?"

"No, that's about it, John. Call me if you have any questions."

"OK, thanks. I'm just going to wrap things up with Dr. Luvkin after you leave."

She came over to shake my hand and said "Good luck," then left.

When she closed the office door John said, "Josh, you can see the situation we're in. I strongly recommend you get out of your contract with Triple X. I'll hold off the newspapers for a day or so. Keep me informed."

"I'll do what I can, I promise." I left Billington's office feeling some relief and also some consternation. The meeting had been, at most, a hard slap on the wrist. My job wasn't threatened, at least not yet. But they also made clear I needed to get out of the porn business lock, stock and barrel.

CHAPTER 23

———

I CALLED HAROLD DWORKIN, BRIEFLY told him about the meeting and that I needed to see him right away, if possible. Thankfully, he agreed and I drove downtown.

"Can't say I didn't warn you," he said almost before "hello."

"How can I get out of the contract and get my money back?"

He thought for a moment. "It's a Mark Twain decision."

"Huh?"

"It's not return on my money I'm interested in, it's return of my money."

"OK."

"If you would accept a simple nullification of your contract, whereby Gabe returns the principal, he should go for it. It would mean he keeps all the profits, which I imagine are considerable after four successful shows."

"So I wouldn't get any of the profit after four shows?"

"Well, it's a matter of timing. He doesn't have to settle with you until they're done. But you're telling me you need to get out now. So you're in a bind. I would just try to get your money out. If I know Gabe, he's not going to cough up profits until he absolutely has to. And right now, today, or tomorrow, he doesn't have to."

"So if I accept simply a return of my investment, how do I arrange for it?"

"That's easy. I draft a one page nullification amendment to the contract, which stipulates a return of investment, no profits expected. He signs and hands over a check. I'll call his attorney today."

"Is that necessary? I mean, can I get the amendment now and just bring it to him? I'm meeting with him this afternoon."

"So you want to do this on your own? Not go through his attorney?"

"Well, I'm sort of pressed for time. If he doesn't agree, you can contact his attorney. If that's OK with you."

"Sure, if that's what you want. I'll get my paralegal to write it up."

With the nullification amendment in hand I drove to Gabe's office. I didn't know what to expect. Gabe is a street-smart businessman and held all the cards. But now, unlike in previous meetings, I had a clear goal. I had to get out of this deal and back to my real profession, the practice of medicine.

Gabe did not expect my reason for coming.

"I have to quit the show, Gabe."

"Why? You're doing such a good job. We're packing 'em in."

I explained the situation, said my quitting as emcee was not negotiable.

"Josh, Josh, pal, you can't do this to me."

"I have no choice, Gabe, I really don't. Let's face it. I'm a doctor, not a cable host. One's a profession, the other was a lark. Can't believe I let myself get roped into it."

"Hey, buddy," objected Stein. "As I recall you did this of your free will. Don't blame me."

"Gabe, I'm not blaming you. I'm blaming myself. So really, no hard feelings. But now, I also have to cancel my contract."

I saw dollar signs in his eyes. I wanted my investment returned. He wanted to keep it.

"OK, Josh, whatever you say."

"Which means, I want my investment back. The 100K."

"No can do. If you cancel, I still have contractual obligations for two more shows, I've got to come up with the money for those shows. I can't return your money."

"Yes, but you've got huge profits from the first four."

"It's a six-show contract."

"What about the offshore betting? Those profits."

"What about it?"

"There's IRS issues, Gabe. Of which I've lately learned."

"Are you threatening me?"

"No, I'm just angling to get my money back. I don't want to have to testify that some Bronx guy stiffed me when the feds come calling."

I could not believe what I was saying. He told me he was afraid of the cement guys downtown. Maybe *he* was a cement guy.

"Josh, Josh, calm down. There's no problem with the IRS," he said. From what Ms. Rachaelson told me I was pretty certain he was lying, but did not call him on it. "But you've got me in a bind. I got no emcee, I got two more shows to pay for. What am I going to do?"

Since Brendan was in the slammer and Gabe's thick accent precluded any audience contact, it's true the show was officially without an emcee. But acts were booked and he wanted to continue. And strangely, I was still attached to the show on some level, if no longer by investment, then with my relationship with Jack Strawn. Then it hit me. A solution!

"Jack Strawn."

"Jack Strawn?"

"Yeah, he's got that folksy southern accent, engages well with people. If I can get him to agree to emcee the last two shows, will you hire him? He knows the show already, the acts. Why not?"

We were suddenly buddies again. I pushed the Mark Twain route.

"I'll make a deal," I said. "Return my 100K, via cashier's check today. You keep all the profits. The betting, the re-runs, whatever. I'll relinquish all claims. As soon as your check clears the bank, I get hold of Strawn, convince him to do the show."

He looked at me and let out a slow smile. "I have his number, you know."

"Fine," I said. "You can call him yourself. But I think he'll want to hear from me before accepting your offer. And who knows what I might tell him?"

Gabe did not answer right away.

"And one more promise, to sweeten the pot. If the feds come calling, I know nuttin'. Nuttin', you hear." Gabe laughed at my failed attempt of speaking Bronx.

"Josh, you make me an offer I cannot refuse. I'll do even better than a cashier's check, which I don't have here in the office. I'll wire the money to your bank. But you have to sign a release."

"Which, as it turns out, I happen to have with me."

He carefully reviewed Dworkin's one-page contract amendment. The key sentence he read out loud. "In exchange for return of said investment, the undersigned hereby releases any claim on past, current or future profits arising in any manner out of the show *Consenting Adults Only*."

"No problem." Of course it was no problem. I was probably out at least 200K of profits, which he would now keep.

"Let me know after you've talked to Strawn," he said. "If he agrees, have him set up a meeting, no later than tomorrow. I've got to plan for the next show."

"Will do."

"Josh, I think you are in the wrong business. You should quit medicine and come join me."

"No thanks. It's really not my calling. I just want my money back."

———◆———

I drove straight to the bank. The money was there. Then I called Jack, asked him to meet me at Melvin's for dinner. He would come for the meal if nothing else.

Over enough food to feed three, Jack listened attentively, always interested in making an extra few dollars. "Sounds good to me," he said. "I'll meet with him."

"Just so you understand, I can't be involved in any way any longer. I am out of it."

"So you're not my agent?"

"Nope. I'm done."

———————

Over the next several days almost nothing was mentioned by the hospital staff about the Pierce newspaper review, at least to me personally. One notable exception was a young surgeon, Dr. Jon Blaise. I always thought him a smidgen immature. He liked to tell jokes, often a little risqué, and then expected you to laugh. I always at least smiled, not wanting to offend him, then found my exit. I suspect others were not so polite, and perhaps I was one of the few people who would even listen.

A few days after the review Jon came to the ED to see a patient. When done with the patient he sought me out at the nurse's station, said he wanted to talk about something in private.

"Is it medical, Jon? I'm really busy right now."

"Medical, he said, just take a minute."

I couldn't say no to a colleague, so walked with him to a quiet area.

"Say, Josh, I read that piece in the paper. I watch Triple X when I'm not busy, but missed your shows. Did you really see people screwing on stage?"

This is medical? I just can't, for the life of me, insult someone, though an insulting retort would have been most appropriate. I had to work with this guy. Like it or not, I had to give some reply without pissing him off.

"I can't talk about it, Jon. Sorry. It's part of my contract. I hope you understand."

"Sure, sure buddy. I'll try to catch it on reruns. But I'd love to talk to you about it when you can."

If other colleagues had prurient curiosity about my hosting job, at least they had the courtesy to keep it to themselves.

At work I found myself more guarded. Before the recent events I always felt people thought well of me. Now I wasn't so sure. My role as doctor was not a concern; you learn pretty quickly if colleagues think you're screwing up. But what about my character?

So I did wonder. I think a poll of ED staff on a single question -- Is Dr. Luvkin weird? -- would have found something like 45% yes, 35% no and 10% undecided. If I protested -- "Hey, I am not weird, I am normal, I have good character" -- that would just increase the yes vote considerably.

At home, in bed with the lights out, I explained my concerns to Barbara.

"Josh, ignore it."

"What, my feelings?"

"Yes. You can't tell people you have good character. You have to show it. Just do your job. You'll be fine."

"I can't help the way I feel. Dr. Siegel doesn't think much of me."

"What makes you say that?"

"She thinks I'm shallow, unemotional, immature. And into porn."

"Why all of a sudden am I hearing this?"

"Because I've been thinking about it, that's why. She likes you, because you have depth, real emotions. She reads me as some superficial sperm machine."

"Josh honey, you are really going off on the deep end. What the hell is this all about?"

"Please, just listen to me."

"I'm listening."

"I've been thinking a lot about this lately. I'm Mr. Straight Arrow who somehow got bent a little with this porn thing, and now is trying his damndest to get unbent. But now there's this image, a well-off young doctor who likes to dabble, make a fool of himself."

"Is that your perception of yourself?"

"No, but I think that's mostly what people see."

"You're losing me."

"That's what they see, that's what Dr. Siegel sees, because I've had it too good. No childhood trauma, no abuse, no want of material things."

"That's bad? Sounds pretty good to me."

"I'm not making myself clear."

"No, you're not."

I sat up, turned on the bedside lamp.

"What are you doing?"

"I want you to look at me."

She sat up beside me. "I'm looking," she said.

"What do you see?"

"A tired, sleepy man who's had a rough day."

"Do you think I'm capable of emotional involvement?"

"Josh, you're as capable as anyone. I just don't get your point."

"I'm not going to change. I am what I am."

"No one's asking you to change."

"The world's asking. Dr. Siegel is asking. My parents are asking. My colleagues are asking."

"Which colleagues?"

"All of them. Silently, with their eyes."

"Change to what, pray tell?"

"They want a different Josh. I can feel it. But I am what I am. Outwardly, they see this competent doctor, but one who acts like Curious George the monkey, who can't keep his nose out of trouble. Did you ever read those books?"

"No, can't say I have."

"I read them to my niece and nephew when they were little. Kids love them. George -- the monkey -- goes from trouble to trouble, but never shows emotion, concern, fright. He brushes everything off, ready for the next adventure. A likeable but superficial creature. But that's not me. I'm as human as anyone, capable of love, affection, emotional ups and downs. Somehow, that image is never projected. Only this superficial one. I don't think Dr. Siegel gets it."

"I get it. I could not fall in love with someone who was likable but superficial. You need to stop worrying about your image. You're not running for office. Maybe you should see Dr. Sobel as a patient."

"I've thought about it."

"Well, why don't you?"

"She's on the staff. A friend, also. Not workable."

"Then someone else?"

"No, I've got to figure this out by myself. Talking about it helps. Your listening to me helps. More than you know."

"OK, I'm happy to listen. But I'm not your therapist. Not qualified. And not interested either. If you ever need professional help, don't look to me as a substitute. Promise?"

"Promise. I'm not an idiot."

"Well…" She held the word longer than necessary, like in an old comedy routine.

"What were you going to say? That you're not so sure?"

"Sorry, I couldn't resist."

"Seriously, I've got to figure this out, and talking to you is all I need right now. I have no trouble with who I am, but do feel a little uncomfortable with how I perceive others see me.

That's all. I am not looking for a personality makeover."

"Well, I like you the way you are. But I don't like to see you so stressed out about your self-image. As the one person closest to you, I am telling you, just do your job, and you'll be fine. Stop worrying about what people think. It'll get you nowhere. You can't live your life for others. I love you, that's all that matters, or should matter."

"Of course, what you say is true."

"About loving you?"

"Well, that too, but not trying to live your life for others. I never have, and I really don't care what people think as long as I'm comfortable with myself."

"Are you?"

"Yes, I really think so."

"Is that a hedge?"

"No. I do keep thinking about it, but don't plan any makeovers. So the answer is yes, I am comfortable with who I am."

"So let it go. Count your blessings. Me, for one. Your health for two. Your career for three."

Our conversation was a tonic. Dr. Siegel did hint on more than one occasion I might benefit from individual therapy, and although I had *thought* of seeking that kind of help it was a fleeting thought. I might change my mind, but now I just needed reassurance from someone close. Once again, emotionally rescued by Barbara. I turned the light off, held her in my arms and we lay back down.

"I feel better already. You're a great listener, you really are. I love you."

"And I love you, too. Can we go to sleep?"

She did, but I lay awake, thinking. My mind was clear. At that moment I could see the forest, the trees, the stems, the leaves. As long as I stayed healthy, did my job well, and had someone to love and be loved by, I was fine. People could think whatever they wanted. It really didn't matter.

I came this far psychologically self-sufficient, and none of the recent events changed that feeling. My adult missteps were stupid, thrill-seeking if you will, but not dangerous and not illegal. Maybe there was pre-dilection to porn inherited from my father, but that's mumbo-jumbo. If that was the case, wouldn't I have drifted into it as an adult, when I had the time and money? But I didn't; it just wasn't part of my entertainment spectrum. I needed the opposite sex in the flesh, not in trashy magazines and videos.

The more I thought about it, I realized there was a silver lining to my bumbling, and I don't mean Barbara. We would have likely come together without the appearance of Jack Strawn and that first date at Joe's Plumbing. No, the silver lining was a growing insight, a fuller awareness of myself as a lover, doctor, human being: a new level of self-confidence and self-esteem.

This insight would not change my personality. I would still whine to Barbara when things didn't go right, make myself obnoxious on occasion, do stupid things sometimes, and feel sorry for myself in depressive moments. But these blemishes would be fleeting. The foundation was secure. With that satisfying thought I fell asleep.

CHAPTER 24

———◆———

I WAS FAR FROM STRESS-FREE. I still had concern about Judy's craziness. And now a lawsuit against me was entering high gear.

Six months earlier I received a certified letter at the hospital. Certified letters to a doctor's business address usually mean something legal, such as announcing intention to file a lawsuit – the so-called 180-Day Letter in some states -- or an actual lawsuit. This was an actual lawsuit.

> Marianne Steiger, Administratrix, vs. Joshua Luvkin, MD, et. al.
> In the Court of Clark County, November 2, 20--.
> Notice is hereby given...

The patient was a 54-year-old man who came to our ED about a year earlier, with chest pain. Chest pain patients are a real conundrum for ED doctors. Do you admit them all? Of course not. You take a careful history, go through a work up, draw cardiac enzymes, get an EKG, and arrange for follow up if you think there might be any heart problem. The patient, Edward Steiger, told me he started developing intermittent chest pains after taking up weight lifting about three weeks earlier. Everything suggested muscle strain, but he also had cardiac risk factors: obesity, a heavy smoking history, and his father had died of a heart attack at age 62.

So while I thought his pains were likely musculoskeletal, I did a full cardiac workup. He had a negative chest x-ray, normal EKG and normal cardiac enzymes. I also ordered a CT angiogram to rule out pulmonary embolism, which was negative. There was no indication of anything acute, or even a diagnosis of heart disease. Still, because of the risk factors I recommended he have a cardiac stress test. Stress tests can pick up heart disease not evident in the ED workup. I even offered him an appointment to our cardiac clinic, which the front desk would have made. I wrote in the chart:

"Prefers to see his own physician. D/C [discharged] with advice to have a stress test."

He died a week later, from a heart attack. He evidently never saw his own physician, never had a stress test (I learned these things later). Naturally, his widow sued. Who can blame her? She doesn't know if we screwed up or not. How else is she going to find out?

I later learned Mr. Steiger had been a factory supervisor at Nevada Tractors, and the family's sole breadwinner. At the time of the lawsuit they had a fifteen-year-old at home. I also learned that Mrs. Steiger has a mild form MS (multiple sclerosis), and this prevented her from working. There were no other dependents, so just she and their teen-ager would be the beneficiaries of any award.

Well, not the only ones. Her attorney, a Mr. George Gramble, stood to gain as well. And I knew he would not stop until he had money in his pocket or lost at trial. So Mrs. Steiger was the plaintiff but Mr. Gramble would be my nemesis. Just as much as I felt certain there was no malpractice with Mr. Steiger, I understood Gramble believed the opposite – that not only was there malpractice but that I, Joshua Luvkin, M.D., was the perpetrator.

Because there is malpractice in medicine and some patients are harmed, the tort bar has a good deal. With enough justifiable cases they can do quite well. The problem, from my perspective, is that unjustifiable cases -- such as mine -- get sucked into the tort machine along with the others. And once sucked in, it is difficult to get extricated without expending a small fortune and a great deal of time and aggravation.

In legal theory, Gramble had to prove my care was malpractice. In reality, because we had a dead patient and a sympathetic widow, I had to prove it was not. I instinctively sensed my task would be harder. How much harder, I would soon learn.

The lawsuit was three pages of repetition, apparently routine in this type of document. The key paragraph stated:

> 3. Dr. Luvkin fell below the standard of care in refusing to admit Mr. Steiger to the hospital for proper cardiac evaluation. By failing to admit and assure proper workup of the patient, Dr. Luvkin is responsible for the subsequent demise of Mr. Steiger...

Refusing to admit? I never refused to admit him. Hospital admission wasn't indicated. Also named in the suit was the hospital itself, as my employer, and an Urgent Care physician who had seen the patient a week earlier, for chest discomfort. This physician judged the pains musculoskeletal from the weight lifting and didn't even do a cardiac evaluation. He told Mr. Steiger to hold off weight lifting, take some Tylenol and return if the pains didn't go away. The lawsuit alleged this Urgent Care physician should have sent Mr. Steiger right to the hospital for a cardiac evaluation.

An autopsy showed blockage of his left anterior descending coronary artery. These things happen. A stress test might have found it and led to corrective heart surgery. But as it stood, there was no reason to admit him to the hospital the day of his ED visit. He should have made the appointment with our cardiac clinic, or he should have followed up with his own doctor. He also should never have smoked or eaten himself into obesity.

We demand a trial by jury, the complaint continued. A dollar amount for the claim wasn't stated.

I was depressed. No doctor likes to be sued, but to be accused of malpractice when it wasn't is a bummer. A real downer. I told Barbara about the lawsuit. She was supportive of course, but otherwise naïve about these matters.

The next day I called my insurance company and told them I was being sued. The case was now in their hands. They would hire a lawyer, he or she would find an expert for my defense, I would be deposed, experts would be deposed, there might be talk of settlement. If the plaintiff won, the widow's attorney would get about 40% of the award. For a man dying of natural causes, in major part self-inflicted, the lawyer could win more than I might earn in several years of medical practice. The tort bar would argue "or earn nothing," but that is a ruse. They earn a lot. Or else there wouldn't be all those ads on TV. And I wouldn't be paying $30K a year for malpractice insurance.

Anyway, these cases usually take one-two years to resolve. I made up my mind from the beginning though, I would go to trial. I would not settle this claim for malpractice, because there was none.

———— ◆ ————

The plaintiff's attorney obtained an "expert's report" to go with the lawsuit. Experts are for hire in any aspect of medicine, both on the defense and plaintiff side. Physicians who function as plaintiff experts often end up on lists shopped around by plaintiff attorneys. The expert against me practiced cardiology in New Orleans, Dr. Michael BonVonJon. His letter was a composite of medical and legal jargon, clearly crafted in part by the recipient.

Dear Mr. Gramble:

I have reviewed the records in detail re: Marianne Steiger vs. Dr. Joshua Luvkin

In my opinion, with a reasonable degree of medical certainty, Dr. Luvkin fell below the standard of care in this case. Specifically, he did not assure a timely stress test on Mr. Steiger. He should have either admitted Mr. Steiger from the ED, or consulted a cardiologist in the ED, and let the cardiologist make the determination.

In my opinion, a board certified cardiologist would have arranged an immediate stress test, a cardiac catheterization, or suitable follow up for these tests, and not let the matter drop. Dr. Luvkin is not a cardiologist, and by his own notes recognized the inherent risk in this patient. Specifically, under "risks" in the ED record he noted "obesity," "smoking history," and "positive family history."

In my opinion, Had Dr. Luvkin acted in manner dictated by the accepted Standard of Care in this case, Mr. Steiger would be alive today. I hold this opinion with a reasonable degree of medical certainty.

> Michael BonVonJon, MD, FACC
> Board Certified in Cardiology
> New Orleans Center for Excellent
> Cardiology

For some reason his letter made no mention of the Urgent Care physician. Presumably Mr. Gramble had another expert for that claim. Though Dr. BonVonJon had not yet been deposed, his position was clear. I was not looking forward to his deposition.

My deposition took place in mid-March, six months after the lawsuit filing, and only two weeks after the Pierce review of *Consenting Adults Only*. Present besides myself were: my insurance-company-hired lawyer, William Randall; an outside attorney for the hospital, Tom Bigsby; a court reporter; a videographer; and Mr. Gramble, who represented the widow. The following is directly from the deposition transcript. In the transcript Mr. R is my attorney. All questions are asked by Mr. Gramble.

Q: Please state your full name and occupation

A: Joshua Bernard Luvkin, MD. I am a physician.

Q: And where do you practice?

A: Memorial Hospital, Las Vegas, Nevada.

Q: How long have you been there, working as a physician?

A: A little over three years.

Q: Could you state your training before taking this job, staring with medical school?

I gave a brief synopsis.

Q: Are you Board Certified in Emergency Medicine?

A: Yes.

Q: Are you licensed to practice in the State of Nevada?

A: Yes.

Q: In any other state?

A: Currently, no.

Q: Dr. Luvkin, do you have any other profession besides medicine?

A: No.

Q: Do you have any other occupation that brings in income, besides being a physician?

Mr. R: OBJECTION. Irrelevant. You may answer.

My lawyer objected so the judge on the case could rule whether the question was admissible in court. Every time the plaintiff attorney asks something my lawyer thinks I shouldn't answer or divulge, he would object. I still have to answer anyway for the deposition, but the objection leaves open the possibility the jury will never hear it.

A: No.

Q: Let me rephrase that question. In the last 6 months, have you had any other job or occupation that brings in income, apart from your work here at Memorial Hospital?

A: Yes.

Q: And what was that job or position?

A: I did some work at a cable TV station.

Q: And what did you do there?

Mr. R: OBJECTION. Not relevant to the lawsuit.

At this point I looked at Mr. Randall, seeking guidance on what to do. He said to go ahead and answer the question. The plaintiff's lawyer smirked, or at least I inferred a smirk.

A: I hosted a show.

Q: And what was the name of the show?

Mr. R: OBJECTION. You may answer.

A: Consenting Adults Only.

Q: And what was the nature of this show?

Mr. R: OBJECTION. You may answer.

A: It was an adult show, with people doing various activities of interest to that demographic.

Here I sounded evasive, legal even. I looked at my attorney for help. He could not help.

Q: What type of activities?

A: Acts dealing with bodily functions.

Q: Such as?

Mr. R: OBJECTION. My client has answered he was host of a cable TV show. Both the hosting job and the nature of the acts are entirely irrelevant to this lawsuit. If you continue this line of questioning I will instruct my client to cease answering and this deposition will be over. We'll let the judge decide.

Finally! Some relief.

> Q: Well and good. Were you engaged in this cable hosting job at
> the time Mr. Steiger came to your Emergency Department?
> A: No.
> Q: So you began this new job, or extra job, sometime later?
> A: Yes.
> Q: Could you explain why you felt the need to do this other job?
> Mr. R: OBJECTION. The other job is entirely unrelated to the
> case. Do not answer.
> Q: Do you remember Mr. Steiger?
> A: Only what I read in the ED record. I don't remember what he
> looked like or the specific encounter. We see many patients with
> chest pain. He was one of many, over a year ago.
> Q: So you have reviewed the ED records?
> A: Yes.
> Q: Have you reviewed the autopsy report?
> A: Yes.
> Q: Could you please read from the autopsy report, the cause of death.

I lifted the three-page report from the table and read the cause.

> A: Acute myocardial infarction. Ninety percent occlusion of left
> anterior descending artery.
> Q: And acute myocardial infarction is what, in lay terms?
> A: Heart attack.
> Q: Do you agree with the autopsy report?
> A: I am not a pathologist. If that's what was found, I have no basis
> to disagree with it.
> Q: Well and good. What is your understanding of the case, how
> he was treated by you?

The deposition went on for another hour, with me explaining the workup of the patient's chest pain, the thinking behind my decision to let

him go home, my recommendation he have a stress test, and every other nuance pertinent to the case.

After Mr. Gramble finished with me I was questioned briefly by the hospital's attorney, Mr. Bigsby. The hospital was named in the lawsuit for two reasons. I was their employee. And they were another insurer to tap into. Also, hospitals tend to settle more quickly than individual doctors, but as an entity Memorial was no more culpable than I was. Which is to say not at all. Here the questions are by Mr. Bigsby.

Q: Dr. Luvkin, you are employed by the hospital, is that correct?
A: Yes.
Q. But just for the record, you are not insured by the hospital?
A. No. My arrangement is that I have my own malpractice coverage.
Q. In your care of the deceased, did any of the other ED personnel affect your decision to discharge the patient home?
A. No. It was my decision alone.
Q. Were you following any hospital policy about whom to admit or send home?
A. No. It's at the discretion of the ED physician.
Q. So, just to be clear, no other employee, and no hospital policy, had any influence on your care and treatment of Mr. Steiger?
A. That's correct.
Q. Thank you. No further questions.

After the deposition I met privately with my attorney.

"So Mr. Gramble wants to focus on my cable job."

"Appears so. He wants what you said in deposition admissible in court, though you weren't doing the cable job when Mr. Steiger came to the ED. He figures a jury will not be sympathetic to a doctor who moonlights on a porn network. I'm going to argue strongly to the judge that it not be admissible. Let me worry about it."

"What should I worry about?" I asked.

"Nothing," he said. "Just keep practicing good medicine."

See? Lawyers aren't so bad after all.

———

Gabe did hire Jack Strawn for the last two shows but I didn't know -- or ask about -- the financial arrangement. All I know is, he was a success. Barbara and I watched both shows on pay-per-view. In conjunction with Gabe, Jack Shawn expanded the bathroom contests to include the category of "Super-Eliminators!" -- Men vs. Women on Week five. The top person in either sex returned for the last show, to compete as Vegas's Top Eliminator. I liked that title. Made it seem "kick-ass" as if the winner eliminated all opposition.

Because of weight differences between the men and women, the contest was based on percentage of body weight lost. The top man and woman weighed in at 425 lbs. and 380 lbs., respectively. She won, eliminating 2.1% of body weight during the show, to his 1.9%. I figured the on-line betting was intense.

We also viewed several more home videos aired on the last two shows. The best was in the style of an early 20th century silent movie where the heroine is tied up on the train tracks, and a train is barreling down toward her. She is in mortal peril. The video was shot in black and white with thick-font subtitles, just like 100 years ago. She yells out, "Help! Will no one help me?" The hero gallops toward her on his horse.

He beats the train, jumps off the horse and unties her. She says "My hero, you have saved my life. Take me!" And he does -- on the tracks! You want to yell out at them, "get off the tracks!" But lovemaking comes first until, at last, she has a glorious climax. "Ah, wonderful," she says. He looks up. The train is now just yards away.

Their half-naked bodies, still entwined, roll over the rail to the trackside grass, safely out of danger. The train comes rushing by. After it has passed we see the couple lying in safety, at peace with the world. Her words are displayed at screen bottom. "My hero!" Then, "The End." The pace is fast, the actors endearing, the sex realistic. It was well done and the studio audience cheered. The video easily won the contest and has now gone viral on the internet.

There were more live sex acts, of course, and for the sixth and final show Barbara made me fast forward them. On the whole, she thought them revolting.

"How are they different from what Irene and Carl did on their video?" I asked.

"For starters, they weren't before a live audience."

"But people still watch it, it's still public."

"Maybe so. But the voting on who's the best and who's the quickest, I really can't take it. It's sex for God sakes. Pretty soon they'll be putting web cams in the bottom of toilets. You want to look up from the bottom of a toilet?"

"Hey, good idea. I'll tell Jack."

"Funny boy. Maybe your heart is still in this stuff after all."

"Maybe you still want to be a pole dancer."

"Josh, can we not fight? I won't bug you about porn if you don't bug me about pole dancing."

"Fair enough." We kissed, and then made love. No cameras, no audience. The way it was meant to be.

CHAPTER 25

———

ON THE FIRST DAY OF spring, at 9:55 am, a sound rocked the hospital, a gigantic firecracker noise. Everyone in the ED looked up, or at the person nearby, as if to ask "What Was That?" Within seconds we heard sirens, then someone from the street ran into the ED yelling at the top of his voice.

"A bomb! The Lindholm has been hit!"

The Lindholm had just opened a month earlier: Las Vegas's newest hotel, a huge mid-range convention-oriented complex, with over two thousand rooms. The sprawling structure is just three blocks from the hospital. What did the crier mean? It did not take long to find out. The Emergency Department's broadband soon began crackling.

"Memorial, we are bringing victims in. Please prepare for full trauma. Estimated arrival five minutes."

In the first five minutes post-boom, the only thing we knew was something terrible had just occurred in our neighborhood. And, since we are a Level 1 Trauma Center, all the injured would come to us first.

Two burly policemen walked in, one carrying a machine gun, probably an AK47, the only model I know by name. "Who's in charge here?" the machine-gun guy asked. "The doctor in charge?"

The staff pointed to me and they approached.

"Doctor? You're in charge now?"

"Yes, I'm Dr. Luvkin. What's going on?"

"Sir, we have a bomb explosion at the Lindholm. I'm afraid many killed and injured. It could be a terrorist attack. We have locked down the neighborhood and are setting up a perimeter around Memorial Hospital. We expect a lot of injured will be here in minutes. We're here to assist and keep you informed, give you all the help you need."

Where was my associate, Dr. Brenda Hazelton? I looked around. She was already with a victim, the first one brought in. I motioned for the cops to follow me. I introduced Dr. Hazelton, said, "We're both working the ED now."

"I think you're going to need a lot more help, Doc. A *lot* more."

Two ambulances pulled up, lights flashing. I was beginning to understand. "Right. Right. Let me make a call."

I picked up the phone and dialed zero. The hospital operator answered.

"This is Dr. Luvkin in the ED. Please announce Code Yellow in the ED. Let me repeat. Code Yellow in the ED."

The overhead boomed. CODE YELLOW IN THE ED. CODE YELLOW IN THE ED. CODE YELLOW IN THE ED.

In my three years at Memorial I had never called a Code Yellow, hospital shorthand for a major disaster requiring all hands. Soon the entire available medical staff making it to Emergency would be under my direction.

The victims arrived quickly, one after the other. The injuries were horrific, more than we could handle. Some ambulances were diverted to other area hospitals, but we still overflowed with people in shock, needing amputations, blood transfusions, emergency surgery. Treated patients backed up in the hallways, unable to take a bed upstairs because they were already full. I was about to contact hospital administration to see what could be done, when CEO Dr. John Billington called me. He was away at a meeting.

"Josh, I'm watching the news. What do you need?"

"I called a Code Yellow and we're getting plenty of help. I think we need to empty ward beds upstairs, so all the injured can be admitted. Let's move out anyone who can be safely transported."

"Let me work the phones. I've got Greg Chalmers (the hospital's VP, not a physician), there, and we'll make sure this happens. First we'll double up on 2-West. That will free up an extra wing. Then I'll see about getting people out to Sunrise and West Desert."

"Great, thanks."

"Wish I could be there in person."

"Where are you?" I asked.

"Salt Lake. Western Hospital Administrators meeting."

"Don't they usually have those in Vegas?"

"Yeah," he said. "Ironic, isn't it? Probably would have been at the Lindholm. One more thing, Josh."

"What's that?"

"You're doing a helluva job."

How would he know? The comment was gratuitous, but appreciated nonetheless. My phone rang again. It was Barbara. She was off work, thank goodness. I did not want her in the ED. Perhaps other terrorists were out there, planning a hospital attack.

"I hope you're home," I said. "Stay there."

"I'm on my way. I'm walking. Will take me about twenty more minutes."

"What? Barbara don't come. We have enough help."

"I'm still an ED nurse, it's where I belong. See you soon. Love you." Click.

Barbara showed her badge to get past the guards and came to work. By now I had four surgeons working in the ED, plus an assortment of medicine specialists, residents, nurses and paramedics. Outside, a squadron of cops stood guard, and another squadron stayed inside, including Mike, the AK47 guy.

"Mike, I need a favor."

"Anything you say, doc."

"A surgeon is off today, named Bill Hartley. He's home. He just called, wants to come help us, we need him. He's afraid he won't be able to get through with the traffic and what he's seen on TV. Can you guys get him?"

"Give me his address," said Mike. I did, and he made a phone call.

I returned to help wherever I could, though by now my role had evolved into more management than hands-on treatment. I looked around. All twenty patient rooms were full, and at least another twenty patients were in wheel chairs or on stretchers. The waiting room was also full with the walking wounded. It was a veritable war zone, or what I imagined a war zone was like.

The TV was on, tuned to CNN. CNN's mobile unit was now parked outside our ED, but the images on television were of the Lindholm's front, a giant cavern where once had been a spacious glass-enclosed lobby. The TV showed two large tour buses turned on their sides, burning. The hotel was now surrounded by fire trucks and police cars.

The country has been through this before. September 11, 2001, course. But also the Oklahoma City bombing in 1995. And more recently, the Boston Marathon massacre. And in the Middle East and Africa, terrorist attacks are all too common. We are numbed by the images on TV, feel distant pangs for the victims, but don't really experience what it's like. It is beyond awful.

A young woman presented with severe burns about her torso, crying out in pain. We had patients who couldn't see, others who couldn't walk, still others who couldn't breathe.

A stretcher rolled in from a just-arrived ambulance. A nurse yelled out. "She's only eight-years old! Get Dr. Armstrong over here, now, please!"

I ran to the stretcher. The girl's right leg was broken in two, with the lower half hanging by tendons. The bone was shattered. A tourniquet wrapped tight around her lower thigh. A paramedic bagged her lungs with a tight fitting mask, to assure she'd get enough oxygen. She was in shock, probably about to die.

Dr. Armstrong rushed over, did a twenty-second exam and gave orders. "We've got to get her to the OR. NOW!! I'm going to save that goddamn leg! Do you hear me?!"

IV's were placed, the girl was intubated, heart monitor attached, vital signs checked. She was still alive. A nurse, a paramedic, a resident in orthopedics and Dr. Armstrong wheeled her cart away. God knows where they found an empty OR, but I knew Bill Armstrong would not leave the girl's side until he had done everything possible to save her.

I never saw her parents. I later learned they had been killed instantly.

Two paramedics pushed in a stretcher holding a dead victim. They used an entrance away from the registration area.

"Doc, you got to pronounce."

"OK, bring it to the back room."

I followed the stretcher. A long-standing agreement with the county coroner was that Memorial's ED physicians would pronounce the already dead and thus sign the death certificate. This was just a bureaucratic chore, but if the death is in our neighborhood they bring the body to us. I could refuse, have it go straight to the morgue, but then someone would probably call the next day and still ask me to sign the certificate. Since it's just a one minute chore I figured to just get it over with and then return to the victims we could help.

"Doc, you're not gonna like this one."

"I don't like any of them," I replied. "What makes you say that?"

"You'll see."

I pulled back the sheet. The man had no head. I quickly replaced the sheet.

"Where's his head?"

"They're still looking for it."

"Name?"

They gave me his wallet. Howard Carrolton, age 47. I signed a DOA form, attached it to his ankle. He would be taken to the basement morgue in a few minutes.

"If you find the head, don't let me know."

"Sure thing, Doc."

The ED filled with an acrid smell, a result of burned flesh, residual bomb dust, and some smoke from the neighborhood. I ordered fans to be placed at the entrance, to help remove the smell. The dead were pronounced by whatever physician was available, then moved to the morgue as quickly as possible.

"...No one has claimed responsibility," the TV cackled. "Police are treating this as a terrorist attack, but so far no clues as to who is responsible. It appears to be the result of a massive truck explosion, right at the entrance to the hotel..."

In the background I heard another siren. This one was a police car, its revolving roof light stopping just feet from our entrance. Out popped Dr. Bill Hartley. Our surgeon had arrived from Henderson just twenty minutes following Mike's phone call.

"You will not believe the ride I just had," Bill said. He was pumped and ready to go to work.

Just then, one of the policemen came up to me. "Doc, they want to interview you. Can you give them five minutes?"

"Who?"

"CNN. They're outside. Told them I'd ask."

"Do they come in here?"

"Probably just at the entrance. They don't want to interfere with any patient activity."

"OK."

The reporter, a woman in her thirties, was accompanied by a sound person and a cameraman, standard procedure for CNN in the field.

"Dr. Luvkin, can you tell us how many injured you've treated today?"

"We don't know yet. Certainly dozens."

"And many have arrived just to be pronounced?"

"Unfortunately, yes."

"Anything about the nature of the injuries to give a clue as to what happened?"

"Nothing more than what's been reported. A massive bomb blast. We've seen a fair number of glass-embedded injuries. Several people with burns and loss of limbs. It's pretty horrific. Many patients have gone to the operating room."

We talked for another two minutes. She was grim. I was grim. It was that kind of interview and I was glad when it ended. I did not want to become famous this way.

My parents texted me. "Just saw TV. PLEASE call ASAP."

My sister Melinda texted. "Josh, let us hear from you. Unbelievable."

I texted back to both. "Am OK. Very busy. Talk to you later. Love, J."

I was concerned about Barbara. I found her with a crying infant and his mother. A second before the bomb blast they had exited one of the lobby elevators furthest from the front entrance. They were far enough away not to be harmed outright, but in a panic the mother ran toward the exit and into a rainstorm of dust and debris. Now the baby was coughing, puking and wheezing. His chest x-ray was negative but he needed intravenous fluid and steroids. Barbara held the baby in her left arm. In her right arm she held a bottle and coaxed the baby to drink something. *Woman with baby. India again. A baby in peril. It's OK, Josh. Come back to now.*

The mother looked up at me. She had dust in her hair, eyelids, over her cheeks.

"This is Dr. Luvkin. Dr. Luvkin, this is the baby's mother, Jessica."

"Hi, Jessica. How are you doing?"

Her voice was hoarse. "Under the circumstances, as well as can be expected. My baby's going to be admitted to the hospital."

Barbara explained the pediatrician's decision to admit, and we were just waiting for an opening on the Pediatrics ward. I looked at the child's ED record.

"Shaun should do fine," I said. I forgot to ask about the child's father. Maybe I was afraid to ask.

After the child went upstairs I pulled Barbara aside.

"How are you doing?

"I'm fine." I saw only fatigue in her eyes.

"You look exhausted."

"So do you."

"Please go home. We have plenty of help here."

She agreed. I arranged for a police escort to our building so she wouldn't have to walk back. Mike was happy to oblige.

I left the ED myself about twelve hours after the blast. By then I could drive out of the parking lot. We were still surrounded by cops but there was orderly traffic flow. Over a hundred not-so-sick patients had been discharged or transferred to other hospitals, and we admitted a total of seventy-two bomb-blast victims. Several were still in the operating room. The death toll – on site and at Memorial – was up to eighty-seven. At least a dozen more were expected to die.

I called home and had a long, tearful chat with Mom and Dad. "I told you not to go to Las Vegas," my mother said. Actually, what she really said before I left for Vegas was, "You should stay in town like your sister." I asked my parents to call Melinda, tell her everything was fine with her little brother.

TV coverage was non-stop the first night, and I was chagrined to see my brief interview played several times. It aired only a few seconds each time but even so I didn't see it as related to the disaster. We learned the Lindholm's lobby was particularly crowded at the moment the bomb went off. The two tour buses had just unloaded passengers who were making their way in to register. They were a segment of middle-class America on a gambling junket.

A bomb-laden truck of some sort had managed to run up between the buses and the hotel entrance. A few people were actually run over before the truck exploded. Everyone in or near the buses, and in the hotel lobby, was vulnerable. The timing looked to be exact, to make the most impact. A surveillance camera showed two men in the truck just before the explosion, their faces not visible. They were blown to bits but body parts were apparently found. Over the next two days we would often hear "forensic analysis is being performed" on the perpetrators. Or at least on their body parts.

———◆———

The bomb went off on March 21. Two days later Dr. Billington called a hospital staff meeting to thank all the employees for their heroic efforts, to report on patients in general terms, and to read a commendatory letter from the Mayor of Las Vegas. This was my first day back at work and I could not leave the ED, so viewed the meeting on closed circuit TV. I will quote part of the Mayor's letter, as read by our CEO.

"The City of Las Vegas thanks Memorial Hospital and its staff, particularly your ED team under the direction of Dr. Joshua Luvkin, for their tireless work during this horrific tragedy."

CHAPTER 26

———◆———

BEFORE BARBARA, MY MEALS WERE either at the hospital, or at home via a microwave oven. I rarely used the stove, and then only the top, for soup or boiling hotdogs. I never once, not once, used the oven. I wasn't even sure how to turn it on.

After Barbara, we used the oven a lot. She liked to cook, which was a good thing. And she liked to shop for food (and other things as well). Her favorite store was a Whole Foods near my building. She would go about once a week. I hated to go. Nothing was in alphabetical order, there were too many varieties of every item to make a rational choice, and I have no feel for what is "organic" vs. "inorganic." If there are organic vegetables, are there inorganic ones? Does one have carbon and the other not? Clearly, my knowledge of organic chemistry was not useful on this subject.

"Don't be so silly, Josh," she would say. "It's better food."

Her meals were delicious. She made me happy in bed, happy in the kitchen, and happy at work. I had found my mate for life and knew we would one day marry.

We didn't always work the same shifts in the ED. She started out on the night shift but later changed to days, 7 am to 7 pm. I rotated much more, some weeks nights and some weeks, days. She would shop on her days off, make dinner and keep it in the fridge for me to eat whenever I got home. Occasionally -- not often enough -- I would be able to come home after a long day to a hot meal.

One such occasion came just three days after the Lindholm bombing. By then the ED was back to normal, though Memorial was still full of blast victims. I entered the apartment, in my usual glad-as-hell-to-be-home-what's-for-dinner mood.

"How did it go today, Honey?" she asked.

"Two more died today," I said.

"That's too bad."

"What's for dinner?"

"Your favorite."

"Brisket?"

"Of course."

I washed up and we sat down to eat. I eat too fast when hungry and started woofing down the food. "It's delicious, as always."

"I talked to my sister today," she said.

"Oh? What's going on in the Pacific Northwest?"

"They might be coming here next month."

"Who's the 'they'? Your parents too?" I had not yet met any of her family.

"No, just my sister and brother-in-law. They've never been to Vegas and want to visit."

"I thought they came for your graduation?"

"Just my parents came. My sister couldn't come then."

"What about your parents?"

"They really don't travel much. Since they were just here for graduation, they won't be coming back anytime soon."

"Well, maybe they should hold off, you know, in case we…"

"Get married?"

"Well, yeah."

"I can't tell them not to come because we might be getting married. I'd only do that if we have a set date."

"Do we have to decide this right now?"

"No, of course not. Just thought you should know."

"Your cooking is great. I'm glad I kept the stove."

She twirled ice in her glass with a finger, as if there was something else she wanted to say. She did not make eye contact.

"Is something wrong? You seem different all of a sudden. Is it because I didn't pick a date while I'm eating your delicious brisket? You know I can't think and eat at the same time."

She didn't laugh. Maybe my comment wasn't funny after all.

"Did you hear anything at work?"

"About what?"

"Anyone say anything to you about a newspaper article?"

"No. What are you talking about?"

"Don't be upset. I hate to be the one to show you, but I don't want someone else throwing it in your face."

Before I could ask her to clarify she got up from the table and walked over to the kitchen counter. She pulled a newspaper from under a pile of folded brown bags and handed it over. It was the most recent edition of *National Investigator,* a trashy tabloid.

"I saw this at Whole Foods. At the checkout counter. I've never bought the *Investigator* in my life. Imagine my surprise."

There on the front page was the usual come-on about the latest celebrity's infidelity. But what caught Barbara's attention at the checkout counter was a small headline in the upper right corner: "Vegas Doc Hero and Porn Star – Page 3." I turned to page 3. The headline stretched the width of the page.

Doctor Hero / Doctor Pinhead

Beneath this headline, a sub-headline:

Same Guy? You Betcha!

Beneath *that* headline were two pictures – of me. On the left I am in front of the CNN camera, answering questions about the Lindholm Hotel explosion. The CNN logo is clearly visible in the picture. The label at the bottom of the picture is "*Investigator*'s Hero." On the right is a still photo taken from the XXX-cable show, with the show's logo Consenting Adults Only prominently displayed in the background. The label at the bottom is "Investigator's Pinhead."

I stopped eating and read the two paragraphs making up the entire story.

> Most victims of the Lindholm Hotel explosion in Las Vegas on Monday were taken to nearby Memorial Hospital, where they were expertly treated in the Emergency Department, under the direction of Dr. Joshua Luvkin. He went on national news to discuss the plight of the victims and the plan for treatment. He and his staff are credited with saving many lives, and their work is ongoing. Along with firefighters, police and numerous paramedics at the scene, the Memorial hospital staff, including Dr. Luvkin, are our heroes.
>
> But Dr. Luvkin has another name, another persona. He is also Mel Hopewell, host of the porn channel show *Consenting Adults Only*. Why would an ED doc do this line of work? From interviews we understand he does a pretty good job as host. But what is on the show? This newspaper is openly displayed in stores, so we can't be too detailed here. Just imagine all body parts below the waist, on display and fully functioning before a live audience. Mel Hopewell – aka Dr. Joshua Luvkin – is our pinhead for the week.

"You had to show me this?" I asked.
"Oh Josh, I'm so sorry."

———◆———

Surprisingly, over the next couple of days I heard nothing at the hospital about the tabloid. The main reason being, no one I work with reads the *National Investigator.* Or, if they do, they were being super nice.

But I had an outside enemy, a woman who would stop at nothing to get back at me for not loving her. Two days after Barbara showed me the tabloid, I got a text message from Dad. "Call me ASAP at hospital. Not operating today."

I called. "Dad, what's up?"

"Wait a minute, let me close the door." Dad was evidently in his office.

"Josh, we got an envelope late yesterday, at home, with a DVD inside. There was a note, it read 'You should be proud of your son'. Mom played it. Josh, do you know what it was?

I knew, but asked anyway. "What?"

"It's you, in some porn show. We could see right through your disguise. At first Mom thought it was a hospital skit. But the note also gave two internet addresses to check out. One is to some porn channel show, *Consenting Adults Only*. It's an actual show! On cable TV. Are you listening, son? Are you listening?"

"Yes, Dad."

"The other internet address is to a *National Investigator* article, about you. The fucking *National Investigator*! Have you seen it?"

"Yes, Dad."

"Josh, what the fucking hell is going on?"

"Dad, it's complicated."

"Complicated, hell! Your mother is cataplectic over this. She didn't sleep at all last night. She wanted to call you right away, I said, no, let me call him today. Do you have any idea what this is doing to her? To us? If this gets in the local papers..."

"Dad, I quit the show. It was a business venture, that's all. It backfired, OK? It's done, I'm through. I've got bigger worries." I immediately regretted the "worries" comment. I was thinking of Judy, and the lawsuit, neither of which I wanted to discuss at the moment.

"Bigger worries? Do you need money, son? Are you in trouble? Are you in with the mob? Tell me. We're here to help you."

"No dad, nothing like that. Trust me, everything will be OK. Everything will be OK."

———◆———

Not exactly, as it turns out. The next day I got a call from Dr. Billington himself.

"Josh, have you seen the *National Investigator*? One of my staff brought an article about you to my attention."

"Yes, I saw it."

"Look, I know you had nothing to do with it, and the paper's just a cheap tabloid. But I just left a meeting with Clark McLaughlin, our Chief of Staff. He told me the medical staff -- not the hospital administration – is launching a simple enquiry into the matter through their Professional Quality Committee. You'll be getting a letter soon, and it's all a formality. I'm calling to let you know nothing's changed from the administration standpoint. This is all between you and the medical staff's PQ Committee."

The letter was in my mailbox that afternoon.

Dr. Joshua Luvkin
Department of Emergency Medicine
Las Vegas Memorial Hospital

Dear Dr. Luvkin:

The Professional Quality committee has met in its regular monthly meeting and in that meeting your name was brought up in regard to two recent newspaper articles concerning your outside activity. Concern was raised about whether your outside activity might impact your work performance in the Emergency Department, and whether the medical staff needed to take any preventative or corrective action. As the issue at hand is rather unusual, the Committee feels it would serve the best interests of all if you could come to our next meeting on April 5 and answer a few questions.

This request for your attendance is in line with our medical staff bylaws, (No. 42-3C). Please call my office and confirm your attendance at this upcoming meeting.

Yours truly,

Clark McLaughlin, MD
Chief of Staff
Chairman, PQC
Las Vegas Memorial Hospital

Dr. McLaughlin never met a preposition he didn't like. I wanted to take out a red pen and send him a corrected version, ask for a rewrite. *Revenge of the English-major nerd.* Anyway, his wordy invitation was clear enough. I would be there. As Dr. Billington said, "it's all a formality."

CHAPTER 27

WOMEN MAKE UP THEIR MINDS and men follow. It's not a famous quote, but should be. Maybe Cicero said it, or Plato. Or just me.

One night in early April, just as we were about to make love, Barbara said, "Before we start, I want to ask you something."

"Oh?"

"I want to have a baby. Can I stop taking the pill? Do you mind?"

Do I mind if you totally re-orient my life with a child born out of wedlock, who I will have to support for the next umpteen years, a child who my parents will dote on to the end of their days, and who will make me look for a bigger place to live. Do I mind?

"Why should I mind?" I asked, hiding my first thought.

"Well, it's a life-changer, you know." *She read my mind.*

"So you're saying we should get married, sooner rather than later?"

"No, darling, all I'm saying is I want to have your child. Sooner rather than later. You will be the child's father, marriage or not. Is that OK?"

"Like, you are really asking my permission?"

"Well, I didn't want any surprises, you know, like one day saying I'm pregnant and you saying, 'how'd that happen?'"

"You've been watching too many movies."

"Haven't seen a film in over four months."

"What if I start using a condom?"

"Then you do object." Actually I didn't. I just wasn't ready for this approach. In movies the woman just sort of announces she's pregnant, the hubby hugs her and says 'Oh, Honey, this is wonderful', and in the next scene Junior is half way to puberty. Only difference here: I was not yet her hubby.

"You know I love you. I have an idea. Let's get married."

"I was hoping you would say that. The answer is yes. Oh, wait a minute, I didn't hear the question."

I held and caressed her and said "I love you" enough times to sink a B-grade movie. She did stop the pill. And I did not use a condom.

———————

There are more ways to get married in Vegas than anywhere else. You can have a full scale religious wedding – Christian, Jewish, Hindi, Islamic, Scientologist -- your choice. You can have a full scale civic wedding – themed from A to Z. In my first three years in Vegas I went to three non-sectarian weddings; the themes were Elvis, the Beatles and Star Trek.

And of course Vegas is known for its quickie marriages, with and without themes. For over fifty years there has been a Graceland Wedding Chapel, where Elvis will marry you (he's ordained). On a moment's notice (well, twenty-four hours) you can order up a Sinatra impersonator to sing *My Way*, or a ukulele player to perform Iz's version of *Somewhere Over the Rainbow*.

Also, like anywhere else, you can have a no-frills, no theme civil ceremony at the Clark County Courthouse. Twenty-five bucks and you're done. And no bar bill.

Or, unlike anywhere else, you can have a drive-in ceremony, as if you were ordering lunch at McDonalds. You say your vows in the car and pick up your certificate at the drive through window. Whatever you choose, you can find the right professionals ready to serve. And your marriage will be 100% legal.

Barbara being raised Protestant, and me nominally Jewish, i.e., not observant, we decided on a small civil ceremony in the Courthouse. We had been living together for a few months, and decided there was no point in a long engagement. Sometime next month seemed doable, considering it would just be our families, and Carl and Irene. We figured on a small reception at the Argonaut afterwards, adding a few close colleagues from the hospital. This plan made the most sense. It was quick and would be relatively inexpensive. There were only two objections, both formidable: Irene and my mother.

"You are not having a courthouse wedding, not if I have anything to do about it," objected Irene.

"Why not?" Barbara asked, naïve in the ways of wannabe wedding planners.

"You are getting married. OK, you've been married before but still, you want something to remember. Not a musty courthouse."

"The Clark County Courthouse is not musty," said Barbara.

"Let me talk to Carl. Don't you dare plan a thing until you hear from me. Promise?"

Barbara promised.

Then there was Mom. Her first words on hearing the news were not Congratulations or Mazel Tov or even Thank Goodness.

"She's not Jewish?"

"Mom, you know she isn't. But we want you and Dad there. And Melinda and her family of course. Do you want us to get married and not tell you? Quickie marriages are pretty routine in Vegas, you know."

"Don't be such a wise guy, Josh. You know we want to be there. We will be there. Is she converting?"

"Converting to what? Oh, yeah, I forgot. She's studying Catholicism. Doesn't like the Protestant stuff. Wants to be Catholic."

"I raised a comedian," she said.

"Well, discuss it with Dad," I said. "We're thinking pretty soon, probably next month."

"Why not a small Jewish wedding?"

"She's not Jewish, Mom." Now I was getting exasperated.

"Do you remember Rabbi Mandel?" she asked. He was, as I recalled, a local Rabbi who did a few Bar Mitzvahs when I was growing up.

"Vaguely. Why?"

"He'll do an inter-marriage."

"Mom, you want I should fly Rabbi Mandel out to Vegas?"

"Don't they have rabbis in Nevada?"

"You want I should look?"

"That would be nice," she said. "For once make us happy."

FOR ONCE? Your son is a doctor, for God Sakes, healthy and happy and productive and decent and law-abiding and successful. FOR ONCE MAKE YOU HAPPY?

"OK, Mom, I promise. Hold next month open. I'll let you know as soon as we know."

The next day Carl called on my cell phone. He started right in with congratulations on getting engaged, then said "Irene told me your plans."

I knew he wanted to talk more but I was busy in the ED, so asked if I could call him back in an hour or so. I assumed he was not working since blackjack bosses don't take cell phone calls on the job. He said sure, call him back. This gave me some time to decide what I really wanted to do. I knew Carl would have his own, i.e., Irene's, ideas.

I called back. "Josh, Josh, thanks for returning my call. So Irene did tell me, and again, congratulations. You guys cannot get married at the courthouse. My wife will object, will not come, and will pout the rest of her life. Women are something, are they not?"

"Yes, they are," I said, with a telephone chuckle.

"So here's the deal, Josh. You guys will be married at the Argonaut. In our wedding chapel. It's nice and cozy, will seat about 100 comfortably. And won't cost you a dime. My gift to you. Don't ask, but I get a big discount."

"Carl, you don't have to do that. The courthouse is fine," I said. "And besides, we don't have anyone to officiate. Neither of us is especially religious or belongs anywhere."

"Josh, you are not getting it. I *have* to do this. I have no choice. So please, humor me this once, and come aboard. As far as officiating, you tell me. You want to be married by a pastor, a priest, a rabbi, Elvis, Frank [Sinatra] or The Boss? – we've got them all. Just discuss it with Barbara. With the Argonaut Chapel comes all the details. One stop shopping. Hey, this is Vegas."

"Oh yeah?" I couldn't resist his challenge. "Any singer to officiate? Vegas has them all?"

"That's right, buddy. Who you want? Frank? Elvis? Bruce? Johnny?"

"How about Pete Seeger?" I asked.

"Who?"

"Pete Seeger, the folk singer."

"Never heard of him. Is he new here?"

"Just kidding," I said. "A guy I once knew. Don't think he made it to Vegas. Anyway, Carl, we are planning on a small wedding, only a few people."

"No problem. I see a minimum of five. You, Barbara, me, Irene and the guy who does the ceremony. You thinking less than five?"

"You sure have everything covered, Carl. I am impressed."

"Yes, but there will be small charge for the reception. I can't do anything about the cost there, but it will be based on the number of guests, which you and Barbara will control. Just five people? It will be inexpensive. And if you want a teetotaler to do the ceremony, cheaper still."

"No, there will certainly be more than five," I said. "Probably more like twenty or so."

"Good, so it's a no brainer. Just one more detail."

"Which is?"

"It's a popular chapel, so I need to reserve it in advance. Just need some dates from you guys, and I'll take care of it. Irene said you want to get married next month. Go home, talk to Barbara, and get back to me in day or so, no longer."

"Carl, I am very appreciative, but don't want to make any promises. I know Irene is strong-willed, but so is Barbara. So I don't want to make any promises."

"Josh, Josh, Josh," he said, speaking like a parent instructing his son in the obvious ways of the world, "I am married, you are not, at least not yet. Listen to me, buddy. Barbara will want to get married in the Argonaut Chapel. Trust me."

———————————◆———————————

Carl was right, of course. Barbara nearly jumped at the news.

"That's wonderful! Oh, Irene is such a good friend. We can even invite more people."

Women lead, men follow.

"He needs dates, though."

She pulled out a calendar. The best week, considering out of town guests, the need for a few invitations, and our hospital schedules, was the third week in May. We picked three plausible dates.

Barbara was now off the pill. If she became pregnant right away, the baby would be born less than nine months after the wedding. This didn't bother her, though.

"There's one other thing, I said. "My Mom wants a rabbi to officiate." This was the first Barbara heard about it.

"Really?"

"Yes. It's getting complicated, isn't it?"

"Do you always do what your mother wants? Why do you even listen?"

"So you object?"

"What if I said I wanted a minister? Would you object?"

"Probably. You have a good point. I'll tell her no."

"Then she'll hate me."

"It's not you she'll hate. You know what moms are like. You want to satisfy your parents. It's just a ceremony and would have zero effect on us, on you. I do think it's a lot more sensible than Elvis."

"Well, we agree on that."

"Barb, lots of inter-marriages have rabbis officiating. They don't bite. It would make my parents happy, although I'm not sure about yours."

"Would this mean I have to convert? I really don't like religious instruction. If I have to convert it's a non-starter. We're back to the courthouse."

"It does not mean you have to convert, or even learn a word of Hebrew. It's purely cosmetic, for my parents' sake. In a Jewish ceremony I just have to step on a wine glass so it breaks inside a pillowcase. Then everyone says Mazel Tov, and we're married. Simple. I'm more concerned about your family, whom I've never met, in case you hadn't noticed. Would they object?"

"To breaking a glass?"

"No, silly. To a Jewish ceremony."

"This *is* getting complicated. We're getting married, but we have to satisfy others."

"Seems so," I said.

"I've been married once. My parents will do whatever I want. They just want to see me happy."

"Ditto."

"I guess the rabbi's OK."

I hugged her.

CHAPTER 28

———◆———

I HAD REARRANGED MY SCHEDULE to attend the PQC meeting, which always starts at 7:30 am. They do some business stuff first, then call you in to the board room if you're on the docket. I knew a little something about the process, because it had happened to one of my colleagues a year earlier. He is from Pakistan, but trained in the US. On two occasions in the Emergency Department he had put his arm around a nurse, out of the view of patients, and made remarks the nurses inferred as sexually provocative. They complained to their supervisor, and the issue came before the PQC.

PQC reviews all formal complaints against physicians in the hospital. They come from both patients and staff, and are often anonymous. After suitable investigation the physician is notified if any further action is needed.

PQC has the power to suspend any physician, which is tantamount to career destruction. Such action goes to the National Data Bank, and is reported every time you apply for any medically-related position. If that happens you might find work at a car wash.

In my three years at Memorial I only knew of one physician summarily suspended: an anesthesiologist who fell asleep in the operating room. One other physician was suspended after a more leisurely investigation, because she was using illicit drugs.

It turns out the Pakistani doctor is happily married to another staff physician, and the gestures were, in his mind, culturally-based and not meant to be offensive. "In my country the girls would smile and wiggle away, nothing," he said. But he well understood the seriousness of the charges, and how it might affect his career.

We were together on the night shift a few days after his PQC meeting and he told me about it. "They listened to my explanation. I explained it's a cultural greeting, nothing more. I am happily married, you know my wife. I am not a sexual predator. I said I am very sorry if offense was taken."

"How many were there?"

"I don't know, about a dozen. You know, McLaughlin, Meringhaus, Armstrong, a few others. And the hospital attorney, Margaret Rachaelson."

I remember thinking at the time: a high-powered group. "Then what happened?"

"They asked a few questions, with one or two acknowledging how my actions could be misunderstood. One guy wanted to know if I ever got into a similar situation leading to an official complaint in my own country. I told him if I did, I wouldn't be sitting in his board room, and everyone laughed. When they were done they said you can go back to work, you will hear from us."

"Well, you're still working."

"I got a letter stating the matter is resolved, and to avoid future incidents which could possibly be misconstrued by women. So I have to be very careful, keep my hands in my pockets."

He stayed on staff another six months, then moved with his wife to California.

———◆———

Memorial's boardroom is dominated by one huge semi-rectangular table, at least twenty feet long; the middle bulges out slightly. The chairs are all swivel, well-padded and comfortable. There is a coffee service on a nearby cart, and on each end wall is mounted a large-screen TV for teleconferences.

Dr. McLaughlin sat in one of the middle chairs, Mrs. Rachaelson opposite. I counted ten people, all of whom I knew at least superficially. I sat toward one end.

"Josh, thank you for coming," said Dr. McLaughlin. In our review last month your name came up from several members, who are just concerned about what is going on. We have no desire whatsoever to probe into your personal life or even your business interests. Unfortunately, as you well know, some of this stuff has gone public, and the publicity has affected the hospital.

"We know you've met with Mrs. Rachaelson and Dr. Billington," he continued. "However, this meeting has nothing to do with hospital administration, only with the medical staff, of which you are a member. It's simply an enquiry by the medical staff, a chance for you to give an explanation. So please accept this as just an informal inquiry."

How many of you have seen the show? I bet some of you would like to be on the show. Bet you would like me to recount every sex act, blow by blow. You love this, don't you, the amazing adventures of Dr. Joshua Luvkin. And by the way, which one of you moonlights for the National Investigator?

I snapped out of my daydream. I had to answer.

"Well, thanks for having me. Let me start by saying the meeting with Dr. Billington and Mrs. Rachaelson was most productive. The last thing I would want to do is harm the hospital or my career. Immediately after the meeting I resigned from the show and canceled my contract with Triple X. So I am done, finished. I think in retrospect it was just a bad business decision. You all know the lure of Vegas. Gamble, win big. I had this crazy opportunity to invest in a lucrative cable show. It just came to my attention, and I did it. So it backfired. I can honestly say it has had no effect on patient care or my professional life. I don't know what else to say, but will be happy to answer all your questions."

There were several.

"Why did you wear a wig and change your name?"

"I didn't want to be seen as a doctor hosting a porn show. It's not exactly kid friendly." A little laughter from the group.

"Did you ever consider vetting the business venture with Ethics?" I looked at Clarence Meringhaus. He now understood more completely what my call was about. Technically the venture itself was not vetted, only my initial contact with ex-patient Jack Strawn, so this was a tricky question to answer.

"Well, yes and no. One of the contestants was a guy I had treated in the ED. I called Dr. Meringhaus to get his opinion – from an ethics standpoint – if I could contact this ex-patient about appearing on the show."

Everyone looked to Dr. Meringhaus. "I remember the call," he said. "My response was, you could make the contact, but I also remember asking if you knew what you were doing." Another chuckle from the audience.

"Clarence, let me understand this," said Dr. McLaughlin. "Joshua called you to see if he could contact a patient to appear on a porn show, and you said yes?"

Ah! A little tension between the Chief of Staff and Chairman of Ethics. Focus was shifting away from me, a welcome reprieve.

"Absolutely. It's an ethical question. He had no ongoing professional relationship with the patient. It was a business opportunity the patient had a right to know about. Do you have another opinion?"

Hands raised up, three, four. Dr. McLaughlin called on another doctor.

"It's always been my understanding that ex-patient or current patient, we should not involve ourselves in their personal lives. It seems unethical to me."

"Well," said Clarence, "ethics is highly subjective and culturally-based. It's not a medical specialty like pulmonology. You have to weigh all issues and put everything in context." He was somewhat condescending in lecturing the questioner, a junior member of the staff. "If you know something that could benefit a patient monetarily, and there is no longer a professional relationship, I see no issue here. I did tell Dr.

Luvkin that I would be more concerned if there was still an ongoing doctor-patient relationship, which there wasn't."

Another hand went up from a senior pediatrician on the committee.

"Josh, how much did you invest? And how much did you plan on making, profit-wise?"

"I invested one-hundred thousand. No profit was guaranteed of course, but I was led to believe I might be able to more than double my investment in a couple of months."

"So you invested one-hundred thousand," said the pediatrician. "And how long are you post-residency?"

"Three years."

"That confirms it," he said. "I knew I should have gone into emergency medicine." Everyone laughed. Another hand raised.

"Josh, clarify this for me, please. You contacted this ex-patient, then what?"

"He agreed to be on the show, and I met with him and the Triple X producer. One thing led to another, and the producer then asked me to invest in the show. That's how it all started."

"But you had a business relationship with your ex-patient?"

"Yes, as his agent for the show."

"Whoa," broke in Dr. McLaughlin. "You had a business relationship with your ex-patient *and* with Triple X?"

"Yes. It was two separate arrangements."

"Margaret, help us our here. Does this conform to our bylaws, going into business with one of our patients when there's been *any* type doctor-patient relationship? Let's put aside the ethics for the moment."

"Well, I looked into all this before my meeting with Dr. Luvkin and Dr. Billington," she said. "I think PQC is getting off base here a little. Nothing Dr. Luvkin did was illegal or against hospital bylaws. Were it not for the adverse publicity, this wouldn't even be an issue before the staff. I'm not a fan of porn shows, but no Nevada laws were broken, and there was no apparent breach of our bylaws."

Smart lady. She put Dr. McLaughlin in his place

Without raising his hand another doctor called out, "So we can enter into business with one of our patients if we want to?"

"That would be highly unethical," said Dr. Meringhaus. "It would cloud the doctor-patient relationship. This situation is different, since there was no on-going doctor-patient relationship. If on the other hand, Josh went into private practice and this patient wanted him to be his doctor, in my mind that would be inadvisable. Unethical, if you will. So let's concentrate on the specifics of this case and not get carried away by hypotheticals. If any of you have ethical concerns, you can always give me a call."

"As to the ethics, I agree with Clarence," said Attorney Rachaelson. "I don't see any clear ethical breaks here. What I see are unwise business decisions that simply backfired."

McLaughlin cleared his throat. "Very well, any other questions?"

There's always a wise guy. Dr. Wells, a GI specialist called out, "Josh. See me afterwards. I've got some alpacas I want to unload."

There was more laughter. I laughed, too. It was a funny line.

———◆———

The toll of recent events showed up in bed that night.

"What's the matter, Josh?" Barbara asked. "You seem disinterested."

"In you? Never."

"Tell me."

"I'm thinking what a mess I'm in. I'm thinking I don't deserve this."

"Now you're feeling sorry for yourself? Don't tell me that."

"I'm not allowed to have feelings? Do you want me to quote Shylock?"

"I read the play too. I don't see you being persecuted. Certainly not for being Jewish."

"So maybe it's not the best analogy."

"How many sessions have we had with Dr. Siegel?" she asked.

"Let's see, since the middle of February, so about six or seven. Why do you bring that up? They've been helpful, and you agree."

"Yes, Honey, they have, but you could glean a little more insight from them."

"I told you I'm a psychology dolt. Don't make it worse."

"For starters you have an ego as high as Mt. Everest. That's always been an issue with you. You're smart and you know it. You're a good doctor, a great lover, a model son to your parents. You're one good man, Charlie Brown, as they say. So yeah, you have feelings, but you can't be feeling sorry for yourself. I don't buy it."

"Not becoming, huh?"

"Not at all. I'm just being honest with you."

"But take a snapshot, Barbara. It's not pretty. Malpractice lawsuit. Stalked by a crazy woman. Trashed in a stupid television review. Ridiculed in the tabloids. Yelled at by my father. Called before the PQ Committee. And I'm supposed to feel good about all this?"

"In case you didn't notice, life has ups and downs. You've had mostly ups, until recently. No, I take that back. Until recently you've had *only* ups. You want to hear about downs? Start with sexual abuse as a child, then go to divorce, and follow that with rape."

"Ouch."

"Look, Honey," she said. "I don't want to rehash all these old wounds. You'll get through this mess. We'll look back on it all one day and laugh. So yeah, I suggest you take it in stride, and count your blessings. And while you're at it, you could hold me."

I felt foolish. She was right, of course. I held her and said no more.

———

Getting pregnant does not take long when you're fertile and your ovarian ducts are flooded with sperm several times a week.

"Josh, I missed my period."

"You're supposed to tell me you went to the doctor and we're having our child. You've really got to start going back to the movies."

"It's different these days. You go to CVS and buy a kit."

"Did you?"

"Yes."

"And? You're killing me with suspense."

"Positive."

I hugged her tight. "We'll name him Gregory."

"Or Melissa."

"I don't care. As long as she looks like you."

"That's very nice of you to say."

"The wedding's still a few weeks away," I said. "It'll be like eight months. How are you going to explain this to Gregory?"

"Melissa will understand. She'll think it romantic. If it's Gregory, I'll tell him to ask his father."

"Thanks."

I arranged for Barbara to see one of Memorial's obstetricians after the honeymoon. Based on the CVS test and the date of her last menstrual period, we would have our child sometime next January.

CHAPTER 29

THREE DAYS AFTER THE PQC meeting I got a letter from Dr. McLaughlin.

Dr. Joshua Luvkin
Department of Emergency Medicine
Las Vegas Memorial Hospital

Dear Dr. Luvkin:

The Professional Quality committee met in its regular monthly meeting with you on April 5, and we thank you for coming
to that meeting. No further action is necessary at this point
on your part, and your case has been resolved satisfactorily.
Please don't hesitate to call me should you have any questions
about this decision.

Yours truly,

Clark McLaughlin, MD
Chief of Staff
Chairman, Memorial Hospital PQC
Las Vegas Memorial Hospital

The Chief of Staff sure does like his prepositions.

———◆———

On May 2nd I received the deposition of plaintiff's cardiologist, Dr. Michael BonVonJon. It was taken by Mr. Randall and Mr. Bigsby via video conferencing, so they didn't have to fly to New Orleans. In the excerpt below, all questions are asked by my attorney. As in my own deposition, there are objections, this time by Mr. Gramble, plaintiff's attorney.

Q: For the record, please state your name, age and place of residence.
A: Dr. Michael BonVonJon. I am 65 and live in New Orleans, Louisiana.
Q: And in what states are you licensed to practice medicine?
A: Louisiana and Texas.
Q: And do you practice medicine in those states?
A: Currently just in New Orleans.
Q: Would you describe for us the nature of your practice?
A: I am a board-certified cardiologist. I practice solo, non-invasive cardiology.
Q: So the Center for Excellent Cardiology is just the name of your practice?
A: Yes.
Q: It is a one-physician Center?
A: Yes.
Q: Please describe what you mean by non-invasive.
A: I do not do cardiac catheterizations or angioplasties.
Q: So you are in solo practice. Is that full time or part time?
A: It is full time, five days a week, and some weekends as well.
Q: What percent of your professional time is spent seeing patients and doing patient care, as opposed to medical-legal work, testifying or writing reports for attorneys?

A: I estimate 90%.

Q: So about 10% of your work is what you would call medical-legal work?

A: Yes, that sounds about right.

Next, attorney Randall had him restate criticisms of my medical care, point by point, an expanded version of what he put in his letter. That was painful to read. Dr. BonVonJon did not come right out and say I was incompetent, but implied such.

I did not know Dr. BonVonJon from a hole in the wall, but from the deposition he was well known to Attorney Gramble. I thought my attorney did a great job revealing just what kind of expert he is: a *medical prostitute*.

Q: So it is your opinion that Dr. Luvkin fell below the standard of care caring for Mr. Steiger?

A: Yes, definitely.

Q: And do you hold this opinion to a reasonable degree of medical certainty?

A: Yes, I do.

Q: But you do not practice emergency medicine?

A: No I do not.

Q: Have you ever practiced emergency medicine?

A: No. I of course have evaluated patients in the emergency department.

Q: But as far as the actual practice of emergency medicine, where that is a primary focus, you don't hold yourself out to that specialty?

A: No, I do not.

Q: Doctor, have you ever been sued for malpractice?

Mr. G: OBJECTION. Question is irrelevant.

Q: Well, have you?

Mr. G. OBJECTION. The question is irrelevant, but you may answer.

A: Yes.

Q: How many times?

Mr. G: OBJECTION. You may answer.

A: Five times in my career.

Q: Any could you briefly summarize the outcome of those four cases?

Mr. G: OBJECTION. Mr. Randall I will continue to object to this line of questioning and ask the judge to strike it. If you want to waste my time and my expert's time, you may continue.

Q: Thank you. Could you briefly summarize the outcome of those five malpractice cases filed against you?

A: One was dropped, with no settlement, three were settled and one went to trial.

Q: By settled, you mean there was a payment made to the plaintiff?

A: Yes.

Q: And the one that went to trial? What was the outcome?

A: In favor of the plaintiff.

Q: So if I went to the Physician's Data Bank and did a search, I would find your name involved with those four lawsuits?

A: Yes.

Q: And I would also find your comments regarding the lawsuit that went to trial?

MR. G. OBJECTION. You are going too far, William. He has answered your questions. If you have something you want to enter into the trial that you dug up, be my guest. But Dr. BonVonJon is not going to answer any more questions about his own lawsuits.

Q: Dr. BonVonJon, have you served as expert before?

A: Yes.

Q: How many times.

A: Several times a year.

Q: How long have you been in practice?

A: Thirty five years.

Q: So several times a year times thirty five years?

A: No, no, that's only recently, last five, maybe eight years. Before that it was rare for me to be involved as a medical expert.

Q: So it's more recent in your career, this line of work?

A: Yes.

Q: Just in the past year, how many times would you estimate you have served as an expert for Mr. Gramble's law firm?

A: I don't know, a few.

Q: More than three?

A: Possibly.

Q: More than eight?

A: No, not more than eight.

Q: So somewhere between three and eight?

A: Yes.

Q: Would five be about right?

A: Possibly.

Q: Dr. BonVonJon, it's a matter of public record that you have served as plaintiff's expert for this single law firm five times in the past fourteen months. Do you agree with that statement?

A: If that's what it shows, I have no reason to disagree.

Q: Have you served as expert witness for any other law firms in the past two years?

A: One or two.

Q: Which is it?

A: Two.

Q: So three different law firms in the past two years, and how many cases total would you say?

A: For all three?

Q: Yes.

A: Maybe twelve. I don't keep a record.

Q: So twelve times you have served as an expert witness in the past two years. Does that sound about right?

A: Yes.

Q: And of those twelve, how many times were for the defense and how many times for the plaintiff?

A: I believe all those were for the plaintiff.

Q: So twelve times in the past two years you have served as expert for the plaintiff.

Mr. G: Asked and answered.

Q: Dr. BonVonJon, what do you charge for your expert testimony?

Mr. G: OBJECTION. Irrelevant to the case.

[Pause]

Q: Dr. BonVonJon, unless your attorney instructs otherwise, you have to answer.

A: It depends, whether just a report is needed, or if I have to go to trial.

Q: The whole thing. Report, discussion with the attorney, and trial.

A: With or without expenses for any necessary travelling?

Q: Keep expenses separate. The total fee.

A: It's about $25,000.

Q: Then any travel would be extra?

A: Yes.

Q: Thank you. I have no further questions.

Mr. Bigsby did have a few.

Q: Dr. BonVonJon, I am attorney Tom Bigsby and I represent Las Vegas Memorial Hospital. Can you hear me OK?

A. Yes.

B. Good. In your letter, and in today's deposition, I did not hear any criticism of the hospital or its personnel. Apart from Dr. Luvkin, do you have any specific criticism of the hospital personnel, such as nurses or nurses' aides?

A. No. The care and decision to not admit were rendered by Dr. Luvkin. I have no argument with the hospital itself, expect that they employed Dr. Luvkin.

Q. Thank you. No further questions.

Attorney Randall's cover letter with the deposition asked me to call "after you have reviewed it." I called immediately.

"I read Dr. BonVonJon's deposition."

"Good. What'd you think?

"The guy's a whore."

"Appears so. But I don't know how much the judge is going to allow in court. I expect she will strike my questions about his own lawsuits. My guess is, she'll allow the part about his frequency of working as plaintiff's expert."

"Yeah," I said. "Gramble will probably just say it shows he's experienced."

"No, I think it will show what he is, a hired gun. But there's a risk also. Some jurors may feel too many doctors look the other way to protect colleagues. They may see BonVonJon as courageous to speak out against another doctor. You never know in these trials. You and I know the guy's a whore, but lay people may see things differently."

"Is the hospital still in the case?" I asked.

"As far as I know. Why, have you heard anything?"

"No. But what's the point? Bigsby has established the hospital played no role, except as my employer."

"Exactly. I did send you their expert's deposition, didn't I?"

"Yeah, the ED doctor from Phoenix. All of four pages. Seems Gramble got in and out of that deposition pretty quickly."

"Yes, the hospital's expert made it clear that Gramble was barking up the wrong tree by naming Memorial. But I don't think he'll drop the hospital. The employer is always on the hook, and the hospital has deep pockets. Gramble will keep them in to the end."

"Let me ask you something," I said. "Does Mr. Bigsby decide if and when to settle, or is that up to the hospital's lead counsel, Margaret Rachaelson?"

"Funny, you should ask," said Mr. Randall. "I recently had that discussion with Tom. He said Mrs. Rachaelson has the final call but she always defers to his law firm, of which he is a partner. And just in case you're wondering, Tom has made it perfectly clear to her that the suit is without merit, and that Gramble is a troll. So whichever way this thing goes, I don't think you'll have a problem with the hospital."

"That's good." I saw no point in bringing up my previous encounters with Attorney Rachaelson. "Well, thanks for your effort. I think you did a great job with Dr. BonVonJon."

"We'll see. The next deposition will by your defense expert, Dr. Davis."

"Is it scheduled?

"Not yet. I've got to arrange it with Gramble. I'll try to get it done over the next couple of months."

"OK. Let me know. I'm curious what he'll say."

CHAPTER 30

———◆———

EARLY MAY WAS A QUIET interlude. There were no Judy intrusions, no hospital meetings, no ED disasters, no cable porn shows, and nothing new with the lawsuit. Wedding plans were afoot, of course, but otherwise life was more or less back to normal. I say 'more or less' because I did sense a subtle change at the hospital. Colleagues and staff seemed to look at me differently, compared to the pre-Triple X days.

"You're imagining things, Josh," Barbara said. "We already had this discussion. I work with you and nothing's changed."

"I know, but right after all the publicity I was just concerned about what people might be thinking. Now they're had a chance to digest everything, and I see a change in their body language. It's subtle, I know, but I feel it. Yesterday Dr. Hixson walked past me in the hall and said "hi" but his "hi" was different than before, more perfunctory. And Jillian (an ED nurse) doesn't joke around with me like she used to. And at the last ED staff meeting? Several people looked my way just to make sure I'm still on the staff. It's there, I feel it."

"Well, part of it I'm sure is because of all the publicity. What other Memorial doctor do they know has been featured in the *National Investigator*? Like I keep telling you, just keep doing your job and everything will be fine."

"I know, I know. But it's uncomfortable all the same."

———◆———

Ever since I saw *Father of the Bride* on TV, I knew I would abhor planning any wedding – my own or even a future offspring's. I felt sorry for George Banks, the father. I know it's supposed to be a feel good chick flick, but "Franck" was not endearing. I longed for simple plans, a simple ceremony. Even with our small wedding – twenty-six friends and family total -- things seemed too complicated. But in truth I didn't have to do much. Carl, Irene, Barbara, and my own mother did most of the heavy lifting.

The big sticking point for the wedding ceremony – would it be Elvis, Pete Seeger or a rabbi officiating – turned out to be less of a problem than I imagined. My parents made the calls and found one Chaim Rubin, the rabbi for Hillel at UNLV. He was happy to officiate a mixed marriage. Barbara and I met with him a week before the wedding. He is a rotund fellow, about forty, clearly in tune with the times.

"I do about one a month," he said about mixed marriages.

"How many same-faith marriages?"

"Oh, maybe two a month."

Two to one, not bad I thought. I really wanted to ask him how many same-sex marriages he performed, but thought the better of it. We went over the brief ceremony, the vows, the breaking of the glass.

As to the dress, I did not go with Barbara to pick one out. She emailed pictures to her mother and sister, and together they decided on a second-marriage model, deep-sea blue, with some frilly stuff at the bottom. To my mind, she would look beautiful in a gunny sack, and if she wanted to marry in one it was OK by me.

———◆———

Mom and Dad arrived three days before the wedding. I was working when their plane landed so they took a cab to the Argonaut, where they had a one-bedroom suite. That night I brought Barbara to meet them. She was nervous.

"What if they don't like me?"

"I like you. What do you care? And besides, they'll love you."

"Did they ever meet Judy?"

"No, actually. And they never met Wendy, either."

"So I'm the first."

"You're the first girl I've been involved with to meet them, yes."

"Wow."

"Don't be so sarcastic."

We knocked on the door and Dad answered. We hugged. I had not seen my parents in almost a year.

"Dad, this is Barbara."

They hugged. "Come in, come in."

"Pleased to meet you, Dr. Luvkin."

"Call me Gerald, please." My father did his best to put her at ease.

Mom came from the bedroom. We hugged. "Mom, this is Barbara." They shook hands. I realized Barbara didn't know Mom's first name. "My Mom's Deborah, but everyone calls her Debbie."

"Please to meet you, Barbara."

"So pleased to meet both of you," Barbara said. "Josh has told me so much about you."

"He has?"

"Yes."

"Well, don't believe a thing he says, Barbara. Come, let's sit down."

The next ten minutes were a blur. Mom's questions were incessant, hardly giving Barbara time to answer before the next one popped up. You're a nurse? So am I. It's been a great profession, we're always in need. How do you like Vegas? Grew up in Seattle? How'd you two meet? Josh can be a slob, don't let him get away with it. Do your parents have grandchildren? You'll meet ours; they are adorable. I love your outfit, the pants and blouse go well together. Where did you get it? Josh didn't want to be a doctor when he was in college. Did you always want to be a nurse?

Barbara rose to the challenge, answering all questions, commenting appropriately on my slovenliness or other sins well known to Mom, and generally affirming what Mom so wanted affirmed: *I can take care of your son, Mrs. Luvkin. I will be a good wife, and one day a good mother. Don't you worry.*

Dad was not half as concerned as Mom. After a few minutes he was able to extricate me from the two women for a private conversation near the window. "It's great to see you, Josh, it really is," he said. "She's a swell gal, and I can see you're in love."

"Thanks, Dad."

"All the craziness is over?"

"It's all over. I'm back to square one."

"And everything's OK at the hospital?"

"Yes, why? Is there something I should know?" I never discussed with him the meetings with Dr. Billington or the PQC.

"I don't know. I would have expected some sort of fallout, I guess."

"Yes there was some discussion. I was asked for an explanation, but nothing came of it. No sanctions, no disciplinary letter, no blot on my record. Nada."

"Great. And the lawsuit? How's it going?" I had told Dad about the lawsuit when it first arrived last November. He had been sued twice in his long career, and both times the case was dropped, so at least he knew the feeling that comes with it and could empathize.

"Same, Dad. Ongoing. There's been a couple of depositions. My expert has not yet been deposed. The plaintiff's attorney got a whore for his expert. I think we're going to trial on this one. I'm certainly not settling. We'll see."

"Well, let me know if there's anything I can do to help."

"Hey, you guys, don't abandon us," Mom called out across the room. "Gerald, did you know Barbara has taken up the ukulele and plays with Josh in jam sessions?"

We stayed a half hour. All indications were Mom and Dad approved of Barbara. True, they would rather her last name be Goldstein or Schwartz, but now having met her they could see she was a sweet, charming woman. I was pleased with the first meeting.

———————

I met Barbara's family the next day. They also stayed at the Argonaut. Her father recently retired from Microsoft as a software engineer, and her mother was a retired school librarian. They had already seen Barbara make one huge mistake and, per Barbara, concerned she not make another. My being a doctor was a plus, I supposed, but only in the sense they knew she wouldn't starve. They probably felt unsure of everything else.

Barbara's younger sister Carla was not so concerned. A tattoo on her wrist announced 'Available', a mistake from her high school days. Carla was a receptionist at Microsoft and her husband worked there as well, in some aspect of software development. (Vegas has casinos. Seattle has Microsoft.) I found Carla more accepting of all things Vegas, including me, than I think her parents were. To her, it wouldn't have mattered if I was a Vulcan, if that was Barbara's choice, whereas I sensed her parents would not want a Vulcan son-in-law.

CHAPTER 31

———◆———

ONE BY ONE, THE WEDDING plans fell into place. I had arranged to take off the day before the wedding, and the week after for our honeymoon in Hawaii. Neither one of us had been there, so it seemed a natural choice.

After three months of almost weekly therapy, we also stopped seeing Dr. Siegel. There is no standard for just how long these sessions should last, but we did not want to start off marriage seeing a marriage counselor; that seemed a bad omen. More importantly, we both felt more secure about each other. Dr. Siegel agreed with our plans, and made it clear her door was always open as long as she was in practice. We thanked her profusely and she wished us Mazel Tov.

Now it was the day before the wedding. Our plan was to check into the Argonaut that afternoon, and leave from the hotel for McCarren Airport soon after the ceremony and reception. Barbara did some last minute shopping and returned to the apartment around noon. Before even putting down her packages she called out, "Josh!" There was fear in her voice.

"What's the matter?"

"I saw that woman!"

"What woman?"

"The one who barged in on us. You know, Judy."

"WHAT?!" I was nonplussed. My worst nightmare.

"I'm certain. She was at the mall."

"What mall?"

"Crystals at City Center."

"Did she see you?"

"I don't think so. I'm almost certain she didn't. But it was her."

"She lives in Los Angeles. What would she be doing here?"

"She knows…"

"…we're getting married tomorrow."

This was no coincidence. Judy wouldn't just happen to show up for a shopping trip in Vegas the day before our wedding. Or ever, unless she was up to no good.

"She's planning something," I said.

"What? What can she do?"

"God knows. Let me call Carl."

Fortunately Carl was not working the tables just then. I told him the whole story. "She's crazy, Carl," I said. "I do not want her to interfere with our wedding. She's a loose cannon. What can we do?"

He was immediately sympathetic, in fact glad to be of service. He asked for everything I knew about Judy – full name, address, place of birth, year of medical school graduation. He even wanted her social security number, which I didn't have.

"Describe her," he said, "I'm writing it all down."

"About an inch shorter than Barbara, about ten pounds heavier. Dark-complexioned, bosomy. Attractive face, hair brown with curls at the bottom, at least it was last time I saw her." I thought of saying "she looks Jewish" but didn't. I would be unable to describe that look if he asked.

"Where exactly did Barbara see her at Crystals?

"Wait, I'll put Barbara on the phone. She'll tell you."

After her report Barbara handed the phone back to me.

"Josh, we'll work on this right away. Better get your ass down to the Argonaut. Go to the security office, tell them you're meeting me."

"Thanks. I'm on my way." I told Barbara not to go out, to keep the door bolted, said I'd be back soon to pick her up.

"No way. I'm not staying here. I 'm going with you."

"But we're not ready to check in right now."

"We're packed, we're going. I don't want your crazy ex barging in here looking for you. If she does you may not have a bride."

I couldn't argue her point and didn't even try. Barbara would stay with her parents until our room was ready. Fortunately her mother had the wedding dress and accessories, so all we had to do was some last minute packing.

We took a cab to the hotel. On arrival Barbara went to her parents' room and I went to find Carl in the hotel's security office. By then he had fully briefed Argonaut's security director, Gil Perkins.

"Let me show you what we have so far," Gil said. "We need you to give positive ID." He entered a few key strokes on his computer.

"First, a picture of your Judy Berkowitz from her high school year book."

"That's her, alright."

"Next, a medical school graduation picture."

"Yes."

"And we have her at the mall, at the spot your fiancée told Carl she saw her."

"There she is! How do you guys do this?" I gushed.

"You think your old girlfriend is the only stalker out there?" said Perkins. "We deal with them all the time. Usually, past cheaters who think they can get back in, and use all kinds of disguises. Or people who've made threats before, and look around for some way to extract revenge. We have to be on the lookout all the time. It's our job."

"What can we do?" I asked.

"First, you'll need to sign a statement to the effect she is harassing you, and is not to come to the wedding under any circumstances. The statement gives us legal authority to keep her away, in case she shows up with an invitation. Which she might, you never know."

"Do I write it out?"

"No, we have one here. Just fill in the blank spaces and sign it."

"This is a common situation?"

"Variations. High roller doesn't want his wife around, he signs one of these. Politician doesn't want certain enemies around, he signs one. You've got to be what we call a Friend of the Argonaut for this special service, which you most definitely are. You are a friend of Carl's and our customer, using our Chapel and eating in our restaurants. We have the forms just in case."

There was a blank space on the form labeled "Reason(s):" I filled in: "Harassment, stalking, and potential disruption of my wedding ceremony."

"That'll do. Now leave it to us."

"We have the family dinner party tonight in Georgio's," I said.

"Your party is in a private room in the restaurant, so won't be a problem," said Carl. "She'd have to go through several layers of security to get in. That's not going to happen. Have a good time with your family."

I was so, so glad I had listened to Carl and planned everything at the Argonaut.

———◆———

That night our two families ate in one of Georgio's private dining rooms, seated around a rectangular table. Barbara and I agreed the seating arrangement was crucial, and designated place names. Working down from one end, Mom and Dad sat opposite Barbara's parents George and Harriet, so they could get to know each other. Next came me and Barbara, then Barbara's sister next to her, and her sister's husband next to me. Then Melinda and her husband. My thirteen-year-old niece and eight-year-old nephew opted to eat pizza in their room and watch a movie. Melinda checked on them during dinner and they were fine.

Apart from being Caucasian Americans with a strong work ethic, our parents have little in common. Dad is a great conversationalist, a trait I like to think has rubbed off on me. He can BS with anyone, about anything. The trick, he says, is to just find some common ground and then be interested in the other person. Religion was clearly not a common ground, so already off the table. Ditto politics. Barbara said her parents were staunch Democrats, and Dad is a Conservative in the Ronald Reagan mold; Mom tends to lean that way also. (I had experience with keep-mouth-shut gatherings. My sister and brother-in-law are firmly in the Democratic camp whereas, politically, I always considered myself an Independent. Domestic tranquility at family gatherings demanded we never talk politics.)

Golf is always a great topic with Dad, but Barbara said her father doesn't play. He does like to fish, she said, but Dad doesn't fish. Woodworking? George yes, Dad no. Bridge? George yes, Dad again no. In truth, George was retired and had more hobbies than my father, who was still very active as an orthopedic surgeon; nothing to talk about there with a retired Microsofter. Still, I knew my father would rise to the occasion.

"So my son tells me you retired from Microsoft," Dad probed.

"Yes, spent my whole career with the company."

"You know, I bought one of the first IBM PCs when it came out in 1981."

"No kidding? I worked on the IBMs. My group helped implement the DOS software."

"Did you ever meet Bill Gates?"

"Several times."

They were off and running. DOS and early Bill Gates were all Dad needed to get things going. Other topics I heard discussed were the cool qualities of Seattle and the beauty of Mount Rainier, neither of which my father had ever visited! Some of the conversation was a bit strained, I thought, but they found enough common ground to last the dinner.

Talk between the two moms were easier. They discussed the wedding, the dress, and a little bit of Barbara's history, which Harriett seemed willing to relate. On the other end of the table, the younger crowd had no trouble connecting. Barbara and I shifted our conversation as needed, up or down the table. People talked and enjoyed themselves.

The food was good, too. The dinner was not comp'd – Carl could only do so much -- and I had pre-arranged to pick up the bill. With wine and tip it came to $1975. About what I expected.

Everyone went to bed full and happy. The wedding was the next afternoon.

———

The Argonaut Chapel is small, tastefully furnished and completely non-denominational. If you want a Jesus Cross or Jewish Star, you have to arrange to have it brought in. We, i.e., Mom, arranged for the rabbi, flowers, the chuppah, the Kiddush cup with wine and of course the glass that would be smashed by the groom. It was a simple and brief ceremony.

"Do you, Joshua Bernard Luvkin, take Barbara Frances Wilson to be your lawfully wedded wife?"

"I do."

"And do you, Barbara, take Joshua to be your lawfully wedded husband?"

"I do."

"Then by the power vested in me by the state of Nevada, I hereby pronounce you man and wife." The glass was on the floor, wrapped in a pillowcase. I smashed it.

"Mazel Tov!"

We kissed.

The reception was fun, too. Lots of food and wine. We profusely thanked Carl and Irene. Not even a whisper of Judy Berkowitz.

Mom came up to us during the reception. "You two make such a beautiful couple. Any idea when I might be a grandmother again?

"Mom, you *are* a grandmother. Forever."

"My son, the English major. Does he criticize your syntax, Barbara?"

"Never." She smiled.

"You know what I mean," said Mom. "Another grandchild. Any plans?

Barbara looked at me for approval. I nodded yes.

"Actually, we're having a baby in January."

Mom's eyes widened and she almost dropped her wine glass. She put it down and gave Barbara a big hug, then stood back to look at my wife's abdomen, to see if it was enlarged.

"That's wonderful! I won't even bother with the math. Let me tell Gerald."

"Mom, don't make any announcement, yet, please. Tell him later, OK?

"OK," she agreed, "but I am so happy for you both."

And I knew what she must be thinking. *How will you raise your child? What religion?* Thankfully, she didn't ask. We would not have had an answer.

Just then Irene came up. "What time is your plane?"

"Ten pm."

"Have a great time."

"We will, we will."

We returned to our room about 6 pm, tired but very happy and very married. Barbara changed clothes, put her wedding dress away and did some last minute packing. A car service was scheduled to pick us up at 8 pm.

At 7 pm Carl called the room. I picked up. "Just thought you might want to know, Josh. Security found your Judy in the lobby, half hour before the wedding. They detained her, called the cops. She protested, claimed she was an invited guest, she was your best friend, all that crap. They had the photos, the guest list and of course your story and statement. Sergeant Nelson of LVPD had no immediate grounds to arrest her, but made it clear a complaint had been filed about stalking and harassment, and if she wasn't out of Vegas in an hour she would be arrested."

I listened passively. The only thing I could mutter was, "Did she go?"

"Gil and the sergeant played the doctor gambit, explaining that an arrest in Vegas would be immediately reported to her hospital, and she'd have to deal with the consequences. I think the hospital threat more than anything convinced her to leave quietly. Anyway, Sergeant Nelson arranged for the Vegas police to follow her car to the city limits. They have her license plate. And, being an MD with state licensure makes it a lot easier to track her."

Yes, that's true for both of us.

"Wow! Great security," I said. "You guys are amazing. Who knows what she was up to?" For some reason I wondered what the ACLU would think of Argonaut's tactics, but at the same time didn't care. If she was a threat to our ceremony, she was a threat to the Argonaut Hotel and Casino, so I rationalized they had every right to kick her out.

"They searched her purse," Carl continued. "The only thing they found out of the ordinary was a can of pepper spray, but lots of women carry one to ward off attackers, so no big deal. Gil's hunch is that she was planning some disruptive stunt, possibly with the pepper spray, or fainting, faking a seizure, who knows. Something disruptive, but nothing we could prove ahead of time, and again carrying the spray itself is not illegal. Anyway, Security videoed the whole interrogation, so it's on record. Gil wants you to feel reassured. After they finished with her, he doesn't think you and Barbara will be bothered any longer. At least not in Las Vegas. Just thought you'd want to know."

"Thanks Carl. Thanks a lot. You guys are amazing." Part of me wished he hadn't called, so we would have left town in blissful ignorance.

"You two have a wonderful honeymoon. We'll see you when you return."

"Thanks again."

I half expected to see Judy at the airport, or on the plane. But we left without a hitch and had a worry-free honeymoon.

CHAPTER 32

OUR POST-HONEYMOON TRANQUILITY DID NOT last long. Late in the afternoon, our second day back from Hawaii, I was working the 7 am to 7 pm ED shift. Barbara was home, with plans to return to work the following day. She texted me. "Urgent. Call home now." I excused myself from a patient's bedside and called. She was distraught.

"I can't take this, Josh. Can you come home now?"

"Take what, Barbara? Calm down. What's going on?"

"She did it again. Can't you stop her?" Her voice rose. I moved further away from the patient care area to secure some privacy.

I knew "her" must refer to Judy, but asked anyway. "What are you talking about?"

"We got a wedding present. I opened it. From a store in Beverly Hills. I wasn't thinking, should have known. It's disgusting. I'm not staying here with this thing!" She started crying.

I could not imagine what "this thing" was but it didn't much matter. Barbara had grown more emotional during pregnancy, and my ex had upset her in a way that no phone conversation could fix.

"Barbara I can't leave the ED just now. I'll be home in just a few hours."

"Then I'm coming down."

That would be worse. My distraught wife in the ED would make it impossible for me to finish the shift.

"Barbara, listen, please. Irene should be off work, can you go there, and let me pick you up? I can be there by 7:30. See if Irene is home, please."

"I…can't…stay…here."

"I know, I understand. Please call Irene, and take a cab there. I'll pick you up."

I still didn't know what the thing was, but knew it should not be discarded or destroyed. I needed hard evidence to stop this madness. "Barbara, will you do that please?"

"OK. I can't stay here with this thing."

"Barbara whatever it is, please don't throw it away. I need to see it. Can you take it to Irene's?"

"The statue?"

"That's what it is, a statue?"

"Yes, but I'm not going to describe it."

"I don't want you to."

"Is there a note with it?"

"Yes. That's how I know it's from her."

"OK, wrap it up, get over to Irene's and I'll pick you up."

"I'm not carrying this thing."

"Barbara, listen. You've got to. I need to show it to Carl, and you need to get it out of the apartment. Wrap it and don't look at it. It'll be OK in the box. Please don't destroy it. Then text me after you call her so I know you'll be there. I just can't leave now, and you coming here will make things worse. Please understand, Barbara."

"OK, I'll call Irene." Her sobbing subsided.

"And bring the thing. We need to keep it as evidence." For what purpose, I was not yet sure.

"Yes. Please hurry, Josh. I feel awful."

"I'll get there as fast as I can."

In a few minutes Barbara texted she was headed to Irene's, and I should pick her up there. I ran out of the ED as soon as my replacement came, said I had a home emergency. It took twenty-five minutes to get to the Collins' townhouse. Carl and Irene were home. Barbara rushed over as soon as I entered and we hugged.

"I'm sorry I couldn't come sooner."

"Josh, she's fine," Carl said. "She brought over Judy's wedding gift. Buddy, we need to talk."

"Let me see it."

Carl led me to the dining room, while Irene and Barbara stayed in the living room. On the table sat the "gift," in a box labeled **Beverly Hills Reproductions. Masterpieces for the Connoisseur.**

Carl pulled back the cardboard top and pointed to the object inside. I carefully lifted the statute, a twelve-inch-tall replica of Michelangelo's David. At first it looked normal, but then I saw it wasn't. Its genitals had been whacked off, leaving only a flat area of plaster.

"Wow."

"Sick isn't it?" said Carl.

"I assume not damaged in transit?"

"Hardly, the note tells all."

"Let me see it."

He handed over a handwritten gift card. In a low tone I read it out loud.

Dear Barbara and Josh. Best Wishes and Mazel Tov. Hope you like it. It's my favorite Michelangelo. I can restore what's missing if you want. Let me know. Judy.

I looked at Carl, unsure where to go with this latest development.

"Buddy, this is actionable. You can't let this pass. First, showing up at the Argonaut, then this."

"What do you suggest?" Carl always seemed to have the answers, and so far they had been the right ones.

"With your permission I want to contact Gil Perkins, then have him call Sergeant Nelson of the LVPD. He's the cop who interviewed Judy at the Argonaut, so he knows the situation. I think he can make a contact in LA and get her slapped with a warrant or some injunction. I don't know, but I think you've got to let the police handle this. Josh, take it from a friend. She's dangerous."

"No, I see that. Obviously. But why would the police get involved? It's just a gift. A sick gift at that."

"Don't know what they can do, but it's worth a try. Your Barbara is pregnant. Do you want this stuff to keep happening? She was not looking too good when she walked in with that box."

"No, of course not. But Judy is ill, she needs psychiatric help. Short of locking her up, I doubt she's going to stop."

"Well the threat of jail might. She already knows she better not show her face here. And you're not going to LA anytime soon. So if we can just get some official warning out there, maybe she'll wise up and stop this shit. It's up to you. I won't call if you say no. But just for the sake of Barbara, let me know if you have a better plan."

"No, your idea is a good one. Call him."

"I will. I suggest you take the statue and note home, as evidence to show the police. Just keep them out of Barbara's view."

"I'll stuff it in the trunk. Thanks, Carl."

On the drive home Barbara was sullen. Couldn't blame her. She was newly married to a guy whose genitals, if not his life, were being threatened by a looney-tune. That she had once met Judy only made matters worse. To Barbara, Judy was not some abstraction from my past but a real flesh and blood woman, capable of perhaps anything.

———◆———

The next day I got a call from Sergeant Nelson of the LVPD. He knew all the details and asked to meet with me. Under the circumstances I thought it best to go the station alone, and leave Barbara out of it. At his suggestion I took several photos of the statue and box, printed them out at home, and also made a copy of the note.

The police station on Sierra Vista Drive is a beehive of activity, dealing with many of the Strip's issues: petty crime, vagrancy, auto accidents and aggravated assaults, the last of which there are always a few on any given night in Vegas. My complaint seemed petty in context, but Sergeant Nelson greeted me warmly and I did not feel unwelcome. He has no office per se; we sat at a desk in the open, surrounded by a few other desks where police file their reports.

"Do you have the pictures and note?" he asked.

I handed them over and waited for his perusal, which didn't take long.

"Some gift," he said.

"Yeah, you can imagine my wife's surprise."

"Doc, you've got some friends at the Argonaut," said Nelson. "I work with Gil Perkins all the time. We try to keep the crazies out of Las Vegas. I think we got you covered on that end, but gifts, that's not something we can control. What do you want us to do?"

His question caught me off guard. Carl had suggested the police would know what to do, so why was he asking me? I didn't want to sound like an idiot, and remembering what Carl said, replied,

"I'm not exactly sure. Is there any way to contact the LA police and get a restraining order?"

"There's nothing to restrain here. She sent a gift. Restraining orders refer to physical threats. We can't restrain an out of state person from sending mail to Nevada. However, we could pursue that with the LAPD. She lives in LA proper, right?"

"Right. So what can they do?"

"I talked to my captain, and here's what he recommends. If you're willing to file a formal complaint of harassment, I will contact LAPD and explain the situation. Since we already have a file on her, and she has proven disruptive, I think they will at least go out to talk to her. Now, honestly Doc, I don't know if that's going to make things better or worse, but it's worth a try."

There was no way I could return to Barbara without some action plan. And I honestly didn't see how things could get any worse, so I gave a go-ahead. He typed a statement based on my story and the pictures, I signed it, and he said he would get back to me as soon as he heard from LAPD. I wondered if I should tip him or something, but then realized he is a public servant and any tip could be viewed as a bribe. Anyway, it was not expected, I'm sure.

"Thanks, Sergeant. I really appreciate this."

"No problem. We're here to help. I'll stay in touch."

———————◆———————

Sergeant Nelson called three days later.

"Good news, Doc. My contact in LAPD met with your lady friend. Two officers went out, as is their practice. They read her the riot act, explained there is a formal complaint. She backed off immediately, said it was a joke gift, and didn't see why she could not send a joke gift to an old friend."

"She said 'old friend'?"

"Well, that's what LAPD said she said. LAPD is tough, and of course I fully briefed them beforehand. They saw the pictures and note you gave me. They know the store, too, because it sells high-end reproductions that some patrons have tried to re-sell as authentic. The store's on Rodeo Drive, so nothing there is cheap. Your gal did this with a lot of forethought. Anyway, they explained that further harassment through the mail – including FEDEX and UPS – could be a state *or* federal offense, and that they were just giving her a warning. Then she acted contrite, apologetic, said she would never do anything like this again. Now she's got a file in Las Vegas and one in LA. Doc, unless you drive to LA and lay down in front of her, I don't see you having any more problems going forward."

"That's really good news. I can't thank you enough."

"Not at all. Glad to be of service to you and my friends at the Argonaut. Let us know if you hear any more from her."

"I will. Thanks again."

I wished what he said was true but had my doubts. I certainly knew too much to let my guard down. She not only had a borderline personality disorder, but was smart and with resources. She had capacity for revenge. Did she still have the will?

CHAPTER 33

———

A FEW DAYS LATER MY malpractice attorney called.

"Two developments since we last talked," Mr. Randall said. "First, I deposed Mrs. Steiger this week. She's claiming her husband came home and told her you were certain it wasn't a heart problem, and mentioned nothing about a stress test."

"That's simply not true. It's in the records."

"Who knows? Maybe that's what he told his wife. Anyway we know it's going to be her testimony."

"What's she like?"

"Nice woman. Clearly devastated by his husband's passing, though it's been a year. Has one son at home. He won't reach maturity for a couple of years. Unfortunately she suffers from a mild case of multiple sclerosis and can't work because of it. I got her to sign a release for the medical records. She says she has nothing to hide."

"So I get the picture. They're economically in the hole."

"Seems so."

"What's the other development?"

"We met with the judge and now have a trial date. January 15, next year."

"Why so long? Can't we get this over with sooner?"

"It's a very busy docket in Clark County. The good news is, the judge has a reputation as a stickler, and she won't let it be postponed. Yours is a civil case, so in theory a judge can postpone for any minor felony case.

Some judges will nickel and dime you to death with postponements. She won't, so put it on your calendar."

"How long do you think the trial will take?"

"Never know, it's straightforward, so minimum of three days, maximum of five, I think."

"What about the Urgent Care doctor? Is his trial at the same time?"

"Oh, I almost forgot. He's out of it. His insurance company settled. So it's just you now."

"For how much?"

"Don't know. It's a sealed settlement."

"What about the hospital? Are they going to settle?"

"That in part depends on what we decide to do. I've talked to Bigsby, and he says the hospital doesn't want to go to trial if they can settle for a nominal amount, just to get out of it. He's in a wait-and-see mode."

"So the Urgent Care doc is out of it. Is that good news or bad news?"

"Probably neither. It just focuses the case for the jury. Gramble's basic argument is going to be you had a responsibility to treat Mr. Steiger so he doesn't drop dead. His expert is going to argue that even letting him make his own appointment for a stress test was a dereliction of duty."

"That's bullshit! I told him to…"

"I know, I know. There's one other thing. We discussed the deposition where he asked you about the cable hosting job. I made it clear to the judge it was irrelevant and she pretty much agreed. She said the details of any job you held after Mr. Steiger was treated should have no bearing on the case."

"What do you mean by details?"

"Just that. She will allow Gramble to ask you to list all the jobs you've held since finishing medical training, on the grounds it is simple work history. He just isn't allowed to ask any details of your job at Triple X."

"You've got to be kidding."

"Wish I was, but she's splitting hairs. Her logic is that a simple listing of work history is admissible, but that if the job at Triple X was not related to this case or your medical expertise, he can't go into it. So when he asks, all you do is say you worked for a brief time as host of a cable TV show on Triple X."

"That's crazy."

"I agree. I agree. It's even crazier because in theory the jury is not supposed to do any investigation, but they're not going to be sequestered, so who knows what they'll find if they start searching the internet. So plaintiff's attorney is going to ask, and that's all you have to tell them. There's two ways to handle this."

"I'm listening."

"One, we let you mention it, then forget about it. Two, in my closing argument I emphasize to the jury that any jobs you had after Mr. Steiger was treated are simply irrelevant, just in case they did any searching."

"What about the Lindholm explosion, the letter we received from the Mayor, can't that be brought up to show I know what I am doing medically?"

"Good question. The problem is, if I bring that in, he can direct questions about other awards you received about that time, including the *Investigator*'s Pinhead Award."

"Son of a bitch. The guy's a real asshole."

"He's just doing his job. It's not as much about malpractice as it is getting the jury to believe something that may or may not be true. He wants to cast doubt on your character. The more doubt he can cast, the more he hopes they will believe his expert. It's a game we play, Josh, we all know it."

I could see that. If I could be judged by a panel of peers, there wouldn't be a case. And I don't mean to be self-serving, either. A panel of peers can condemn as well as exonerate. At least they'd know medicine. But in our system, Gramble was allowed to go out and find eight lay people, then try to convince them the widow deserves a windfall because her husband ate a lot and smoked. And he's allowed to omit the fact he will take a large percentage of any award.

"How much are they asking for?"

"The demand is one million."

"Could the jury award more?"

"Anything is possible, but I don't see punitive damages here."

"Could it be less?"

"Could be. If you lose, your name goes to the data bank."

"Well that's true if I settle as well."

"Correct."

"I understand with my policy I can refuse to settle, is that right? And demand a trial?"

"Yes, I checked with the insurance company. You can refuse to settle."

"What are you recommending?"

"Right now, hold tight. Gramble is going to depose our defense expert next week. Let me see how that goes, then we'll talk again."

I badly wanted to be free of this aggravation, but resigned myself to wait. I certainly wasn't going to settle.

———◆———

One morning in late May I was working the day shift, treating an elderly man for pneumonia. The ED was relatively quiet. Barbara was off work, at home writing thank you notes.

The EMS radio cackled. "Suicide at Paris Las Vegas, bottom of Eiffel Tower. We're bringing her in. Check local channel for more info."

In a minute both TVs in the ED were turned to the local channel. The TV news anchor was in his studio interviewing a reporter on the scene.

"Heidi, what do we know?"

"An unidentified woman fell to her death just a little while ago, from the Eiffel Tower in front of The Paris Las Vegas Hotel." The camera view went from a draped sheet near the sidewalk to a point on the tower about 100 feet up. "Witnesses say they saw her climb out onto the girders, then jump. How she got outside the structure is still being investigated. The tower as you can see is some 540 feet high, and at the top is a sealed observation area. Her jumping point was lower down, just here, at what's known as the Experience Deck." The camera zoomed in on the protruding square section of the tower, ten stories off the ground. "Police estimate she died instantly. The body's going to be taken to Memorial Hospital for official pronouncement and an autopsy by the coroner."

"Do we know who she is, her name, age?"

"The police say she is a Caucasian woman, in early to mid-30s, well-dressed. But as to her name, not at this point. Police state they found a lengthy suicide note on her person, but all information is being withheld pending notification of next of kin."

"Was she alone, Heidi? Was she with anyone?"

"Witnesses say she was alone. The area from which she jumped is just above a restaurant and some shops. We understand it does not have an outside observation deck, but apparently she was able to reach the external skeleton and jump. We should learn more in the next hour."

"OK, thanks Heidi. We'll check back with you soon. In other news today…"

I was all but certain it was Judy. Everything fit. The personality disorder. Being kicked out of the Argonaut. LAPD's threat of arrest if she used the mail to harass me. And the need to make a dramatic, final statement, both physical and written. I knew her "lengthy suicide note" would blame me, besmirch my name with its run-on paranoid accusations. From the news I also knew the police had the note, so there was nothing I could do but anticipate more "damage control."

I felt glad to be rid of her, just wished there was no note. The note! The goddamned note! It would lead, I knew, to more tabloid articles. I could write the *Investigator*'s headlines: *Investigator's Pinhead Gored by Jilted Lover.* Or worse: *Suicide's Ex Pronounces her Dead: Good Riddance!*

When the contents of the note got out – and it always does, these things never stay hidden – what would my colleagues think of me then? *That Triple X episode was no fluke. Dr. Luvkin is a Jekyll and Hyde.* I shuddered at the coming onslaught of more bad publicity and was beside myself with anxiety. Any more defense would simply ring hollow. Now, I might be kicked off the medical staff. Judy knew this of course, and planned her death well.

Twenty minutes later the ambulance arrived with her body. Before the coroner's autopsy -- which would be performed at Memorial -- a physician had to pronounce her. Just my luck it had to be me. Maybe I could destroy the note before it was made public. Destruction of evidence would be a felony offense, and of course I would be found out, prosecuted, kicked off the medical staff. Judy would love it; from her perch in Hell she would laugh out loud.

They put the stretcher in the room for dead people. The same room where I pronounced the headless man.

A policeman stood beside the cart, his face turned away.

"Do your thing, Doc. It's pretty gruesome. She hit hard."

I pulled the sheet back and stared.

"It's not her!"

"What?" He turned around. My comment made no sense to him. "It's not who, Doc?"

"I mean, I mean, I thought it was a movie actress, I thought the TV reporter said she was a movie star. But I don't recognize her. Do you know her name?"

"Nah. There's a suicide note, already sent to the coroner. You got to pronounce her as Jane Doe. We'll do the rest."

I was so relieved! The suicide note would not have my name besmirched in a thicket of anger and revenge. At the same time, I also felt a little unhappy the corpse was *not* Judy Berkowitz.

CHAPTER 34

———◆———

A WEEK LATER, BARBARA'S CELL phone rang around 11 pm, waking us both up. She glanced at the phone. "It's Irene." Barbara got out of bed and walked to the window to assure good reception.

"What's the matter Irene?" I could only hear Barbara's half of the conversation.

"What?…Oh my God!…Oh, that's awful…Now?…Yes, yes, of course. I'll call downstairs, tell them you're coming." Barbara clicked off the phone and returned to bed.

"I'm afraid to ask," I said.

"She had a big fight with Carl. He threatened her. She's afraid to stay home. Just wants to come over here until things are straightened out. What could I say? I assumed you wouldn't object."

"Of course not. What was the fight about? Did she say?"

"He's screwing other women."

———◆———

Irene arrived around 11:30 with a small suitcase. She was disheveled, hair uncombed, no makeup. These things did not make her un-pretty, just sad-looking. I instantly felt sorry for her.

"I'm so sorry to intrude like this, I just didn't know where to go. I suppose I should have gone to a hotel."

"Nonsense," shot back Barbara. "You can sleep here on the couch. Do you want to talk about it?"

Part of me wanted to hear the story and the other part wanted to return to sleep. I did have to work in the morning.

Irene began sobbing. Barbara put an arm around her, led her to the couch. "It's OK, it's OK." She rubbed Irene's shoulders.

"Can I get you something to drink?" I asked. "Are you hungry?"

"No…I'm fine." Then she burst out crying and repeated. "I know it's over…It's over…It's over."

"What happened?"

Irene opened the suitcase and removed a brown envelope. "I got this in the mail today."

Barbara opened the envelope. Inside were five 9" x 11" glossies. They did not appear to be original photos, but stills from a video. We looked at them one at a time, not out of prurient interest but to assure it was Carl in each picture. Carl with his dick in the mouth of a woman not his wife. Carl's head between the legs of the same woman. And then one each showing positions Carl and Irene had captured in video, though the female was clearly not his wife.

"How did you get these? Who sent them to you?"

"There's a note inside."

Sure enough, inside we found an index card. In handwritten letters: "Your hubby is a prick. Just thought you should know."

"It's not signed."

"She's a dancer at the Argonaut. I've met her."

"Why would she do something like this?" I asked, quickly realizing "this" could refer to the act or the message. "I mean, if she messed around with Carl, why would she send *you* these pictures? I would think she might want to blackmail Carl."

Barbara had the answer. "Probably got into a fight with Carl, mailed Irene the pictures to break up his marriage, make him miserable. Blackmail is illegal. This isn't."

Irene's sobbing subsided. She seemed relieved to share this injustice with friends.

"How do we know these pictures are even current?" I asked. "They could have been taken anytime."

Irene pointed to a bracelet on Carl's left wrist in one of the pictures. "I gave him that bracelet for his birthday six months ago."

"Oh. So you confronted him with this?"

She nodded.

"Then why would *he* become threatening?" I asked. "I think he would be embarrassed, apologetic. Why threaten you?" I sensed this was becoming more like an inquest than the soothing of a friend's anguish.

Irene looked at Barbara, as if my wife had the answer. But Barbara was just as puzzled. Then in a mixture of tears and words, Irene cried out, "Because I told him about me and Gabe!"

"Oh, no," I whispered.

"Irene! What do you mean?" asked Barbara.

"He got me so angry, I blurted out I had sex with Gabe Stein."

"You did?"

"Just once."

"When? Why?"

"Couple weeks after the video came out. I went to pick up a royalty check. He asked me about one of the positions. He said it was not humanly possible. He sort of challenged me, wanted me to show him. We went into the video room. Next thing, I know, he's inside me. I didn't stop him."

"It's on video too?"

"No. No one else was there. I never would have said anything, but Carl just got me so angry. Right after I told him, he flew into a rage."

"Talk about double standard," I said in a low voice.

"Said he would kill the kike. And me with him. That's when I called you."

Carl anti-Semitic? Who would of thought? Actually, I was not all that surprised. The irony is that Carl had been super nice to me and Barbara, extremely helpful on several occasions, and I had actually grown fond of him. He was a good guy to know in Vegas, and I felt genuinely sorry over Irene's tale.

We didn't know what more to say, or at least I didn't. I begged off and went to bed, explaining I had to get up early. Barbara stayed with Irene another hour, commiserating in the way only an old friend can.

I left for the hospital in the morning, with Barbara and Irene still sleeping. When I returned home in the evening, Irene was gone.

"Went home to Seattle," said Barbara. "I'm afraid she's right."

"What do you mean?"

"It's all over between them."

The pattern was inescapable. I had closely associated with three women since moving to Vegas, two as lovers and one as friend. All were married at one time, with none of the marriages lasting more than two years. The hubbies cheated on them. Yes, one woman was crazy and the other an exhibitionist, so you might say they deserved it. But Barbara was neither, her pole dancing notwithstanding, although I see there might be some argument about the exhibitionist part.

So there was a pattern, but what did it mean for our future? Was I destined to cheat on Barbara? Unlikely, as she was everything I ever wanted. Would she succumb to whatever inner need led her to pole dance, and attract another unsavory man? I sure hoped not. The therapy sessions certainly gave us reason to be optimistic.

Then it hit me. "Barbara, this is not a healthy place."

"What do you mean?"

"Vegas. We need to get out. It's not healthy here."

Was this an epiphany? Yes, it was. Suddenly my eyes opened and I saw what was hidden just moments before. It wasn't just the recent revelation about Irene and Carl, but a litany of things: the malpractice suit, Judy's craziness, the cable show fiasco, the hospital inquests, the intrusion of lawyers into my life and, lately, all the second glances from colleagues and co-workers. It was time to relocate.

"Where do you want to go?"

"I don't know. Let's look at a map."

CHAPTER 35

———

VEGAS IS ALWAYS FULL OF surprises. Two nights after Irene's call the phone woke me again. It was one in the morning and this time Jack Strawn was on the line. He had my personal cell phone number.

"You sittin' down, doc?"

"In bed, as a matter of fact. What's going on, Jack?" I sensed he was in some sort of trouble.

"We was raided tonight."

"Oh, no."

"Oh, yes. The place must have been infiltrated by the feds and the state. Fucking storm troopers."

"So the gambling is illegal, after all? Is that why you were raided?"

"Don't know shit about that. But I do know they busted us. Both the feds and Nevada State Troopers. Coordinated teams. Can you believe it? Ten of 'em. Two guys were already in the audience, then eight more came barging in. Fucking nightmare. I was in the john."

"It makes sense, now that I think about it, Jack. You said the owner never paid any taxes."

"You mean Joe Calabane?"

"Yeah, that guy. The one who runs the place."

"Maybe so, but why what the fuck does that have to do with me?"

"So what happened?"

"I heard people yelling. I pulled my pants up and came out to see what was going on. Got the drift right away and made for the back exit.

Guy was there with a machine gun, turned me right around. Can you believe this shit?"

"Then what happened?"

"They handcuffed old man Joe right in front of everybody. Led him away."

"Where are you? Not in jail, I hope."

"Unfortunately, yes. Which is why I'm calling."

"Oh?"

"I need a big favor."

"What?"

"Can you bail me out?"

"Bail you out!? What are you arrested for?"

Barbara, awake by now, said "Is he in jail?"

"Yeah," I whispered.

"They arrested all the contestants," Jack said.

"The audience, too?"

"No, they let 'em go. Just Joe, his guys, and us. Now they got fat guys in jail. Can you believe this shit?"

Why am I the only one he can call? A wife, a brother, Gabe?

"Did you call Gabe?"

"No. After the shows were done, he said there was some legal things he had to take care of, he'd get back to me. Never did. I called twice and he never returned my calls."

"Maybe he's got his own problems. Did Gabe ever pay you?"

"Oh, yeah, I got paid. But the money's gone. My next paycheck is a week away."

"How much do you need?"

"It's $2500."

"This is new to me, Jack. How exactly do I do arrange bail? Do they take credit cards?" I expected a firm no.

"Yeah, they do."

"Really? Can I do it online?"

"Yep. That's how they do it nowadays. I have the website. I got to read it out to you so there's no confusion."

"OK, give it to me." I wrote down the website.

"Jack, I'm working tomorrow morning, but if I do this we got to meet and talk, fair enough?"

"Anything you say. I just got to get out of this hell hole. The fucking toilet doesn't fit."

It was one of those situations where you just can't say no and still live with yourself. Still, even though bail could be posted online didn't mean it would work. I envisioned being up all night fiddling with a balky website and 404 code errors.

"Is there someone I can talk to who will confirm this works, so you can get out and I can go back to sleep?"

"Right here, Doc. He'll stay on the phone while you pay. Very accommodating. They got to ask you some questions anyway."

"OK, I'll do it. But I need to meet with you tomorrow right after work, to discuss this. Can I come by, say 7:30?"

"Anything you say, Doc. Just get me out of this hell hole."

Officer Pritchett was actually quite nice. Apparently online bail was common. He was so helpful I wondered if he got some sort of commission for handling the call. I found the website, entered the information Pritchett gave me (Jack's prison number, a few other items), and then my card info. The amount of bail pre-loaded at $2500, just as Jack said. Before I clicked "Submit" there was a warning.

If your client does not appear in court on the appointed date and there is no court-approved excuse, this bail is FORFEITED.

I clicked "Submit," and went back to sleep. Officer Pritchett promised to call me if there was any problem. There were no more calls so I assumed Jack was released and went home. It occurred to me his car must still be at Joe's Plumbing Supplies and he would have to find some way home. But there was nothing more I could do.

The next day, by text message, Jack confirmed he was home. After work I drove to pick him up. On the way I cruised by the Las Vegas Detention Center on Stewart Avenue, curious to see what it looks like. The building is a twelve-story multi-sectioned box-like structure with narrow horizontal windows. It looks like, well, a jail. I was glad I could bail him out online.

This was my second trip to Jack's abode, though I never made it inside. He lived in a trailer park in North Vegas, in one of those small units that stay in place, never move. After my conversation with him the night before, I wondered if the trailer's toilet fit.

I honked and he came right out, got in the car.

"I owe you big time, Doc. You saved my ass."

"How long did it take after I did the credit card thing?"

"Fifteen minutes. They didn't want me in there any more than I wanted to stay. You know what one guard said as I was leaving?"

"What?"

"Now we'll have enough food for the other inmates."

"Wow, what a rude comment."

"Shithole of a place. I was constipated the whole four hours I was there."

I was no longer interested in his bowel habits and changed the subject.

"How'd you get home?"

"Cab. My last twenty."

"Where's your car?"

"Still at Joe's Plumbing. I was hoping you could drop me there."

"OK, but something to eat first?" I already told Barbara I wouldn't be home for supper.

"Great idea."

"Where do you want to go?"

"Let's go to The Greasy Spoon. It's on the way to Joe's."

He directed me to the diner. The Greasy Spoon does not have Melvin's quiet ambience but its menu is wide ranging and the food in ample proportions. I didn't want to worry him with expenses at this point and made it clear I was paying. He didn't object.

Over eggs and ham I asked, "OK, Jack, what the hell is going on?"

"What do you mean?"

"Just level with me. Do you have a real job?"

"Yeah, I told you, I manage an apartment building in Summerlin."

"But you didn't work today?"

"Nah, I called in sick. They have a backup."

"Have you ever been busted before?"

"Hey doc, I just left the jail. Did they send you to do more investigation? Why are you meeting with me?"

"I'm just trying to protect my investment in you. I don't get a bail request every night. And I really don't know all that much about you. I just thought this was an opportunity to learn more."

"You know enough. I was married once, no kids. Started eatin' myself to death about ten years ago. When I was twenty-five I weighted 180 lbs. Can you believe it?"

"I believe it. How much they got against you?"

"One prior charge. Aggravated assault."

"Who'd you assault?"

"My ex."

"Oh? Did you serve time?"

"A year. She was pretty beat up. But I'm clean since. No more of that shit."

"She's alive?"

"I assume. Somewhere in Georgia."

"Jack, how bad is this?"

"This what?"

"This. The arrest, the rap, the charges, the whole shebang."

"Shit, I don't know. The IRS got my name. They got Joe's books. There's this fucking Nevada Gaming Commission. Who the fuck knows?" Without Barbara around, Jack felt free to use all the four letter words.

"Did you pay taxes on the winnings at Joe's?"

"No, of course not."

"Did you ever pay taxes, file an income tax return?

"Yeah, five years ago."

"Your Summerlin job, don't you get a W-2 Statement?"

"Nah, it's all under the table."

"Well, do you have a lawyer?"

"Yeah, Mr. State Public Defender. These guys probably make less than I do. Good luck with that."

I felt sorry for Jack Strawn. Once almost a porn show star, now he was in deep legal and financial trouble. And I felt sorry for me. I figured there was a 50-50 chance he would appear in court. No, make it 20-80.

"Where will you go?" I asked.

"What do you mean, where will I go?"

"I don't know what I mean."

"You worried about your money?"

"Of course."

"Hey doc, you're my friend. You'll get your money back. I ain't goin' nowhere."

"You think it's time to lose some weight?" This was, I realized, an awkward question just as he was consuming six eggs and a loaf of toast.

"You always come back to my weight, Doc."

"I'm sorry, it's a medical thing. I shouldn't keep bugging you."

"I got a lot on my plate." He looked at his eggs. "I mean my real fucking plate."

"I understand."

I took him to his car at the strip mall. It was an old beat-up Pontiac. As he got out of my car I said, "You'll stay in touch, let me know what's happening? You have my number."

"Will do."

I waited to make sure his car started, then drove home.

———————

We could have pulled up a map on the internet but I wanted a paper view of the country, like when I was a kid. You just don't get the same perspective from a computer screen. The day after my meeting with Strawn I got a large U.S. map from AAA. I spread the map out on the kitchen table so we could quickly survey coast to coast. Barbara and I poured over it like children in a candy store.

"Seattle is magnificent," I said, "you'd be close to your parents."

"Keep looking," Barbara said. "And let's leave out the Midwest, unless you want to be close to yours."

"Nope, it's got to be west of the Mississippi."

"How about California? Great weather."

"How about high taxes and traffic?" I shot back. "I can do without those. And there's always a drought. I like to take showers."

"OK, Arizona."

"More desert? If we're going to move I want trees."

"Texas?"

"I like Texas," I said. "Dallas, Houston, San Antonio, take your pick. They're all boom towns. We should have no trouble getting licenses and jobs."

While she scanned the lone star state my eyes drifted to Wyoming. I pointed to the state's northwest corner. "Barbara, here's where I spent one magical summer."

She lowered her head to see the labeling. "Yellowstone?"

"Yeah."

"You'd have to be veterinarian to work there, Honey. Isn't the park closed in the winter?"

"Most of it, yeah. Just dreaming."

Then my eye drifted northward to Montana and I pointed. "But this place is open. Bozeman. And it's close to Yellowstone."

"I thought you didn't like cold."

"I don't. But I grew up in cold, and summers are so pleasant in the northern climes. It would be nice to raise our child in a small city, away from this place."

"You make it sound inviting."

On July 4th we flew to Bozeman, Montana to interview for jobs and look at real estate. A part time ED job was available in their regional hospital, and I could make it full time if I was willing to do some urgent care as well. Frankly this was appealing, to have some of my work less intense than a full-scale scale ED.

Barbara had no trouble finding a nursing job in the hospital. We liked the town and looked forward to moving. We bought a small bungalow close to the hospital. It came already furnished, which was a big plus. I arranged to have a burglar alarm installed before our move. The previous owners said they never felt the need. Maybe so, but I would be working some nights at the hospital, leaving Barbara alone with the baby; under the circumstances a home alarm seemed prudent.

While in Bozeman I also made enquiry about a Free Clinic, and learned there was one and that openings were always available for volunteers. I volunteered for a couple of days a month, when I was not in the ED.

Barbara was skeptical of my motive. "You're not the volunteering type."

"Oh? What type is that?"

"Honey, I'm not being critical, I just never thought of you as someone to volunteer their time."

"Maybe I saw too much 'gimme gimme' in Vegas."

"So you're trying to atone?"

"It's the right thing to do. I don't know why. It just is something I want to do."

"So who's this for, the patients or Dr. Luvkin?"

"A little bit of both. Is that so bad?"

"Josh, it's wonderful. Wish I could join you. But with Melissa on the way, I'm going to be super busy."

Oh, I forgot to mention. The ultrasound showed we were having a girl.

I made one other decision in Montana: to buy a gun. I didn't even think about it until we got there. Billboards everywhere advertised firearms, Montana's "Carry and Conceal policy" and "Your 2nd Amendment Right." If an alarm system offered some measure of protection against an intruder, might not a gun offer an additional layer? I had seen enough gunshot wounds to know this was often not true. The victim was far more likely to be a family member shot by accident or intention. Still, I decided to buy a gun on our return to Las Vegas, and learn to use it before we moved.

The only drawback to relocating to Bozeman, and a minor one as it turned out, was the standard hospital medical staff application. "In the past ten years have you been sued for malpractice? If so, provide full details on a separate sheet." My malpractice case was on-going, but I figured one lawsuit shouldn't matter much. It's an occupational hazard, particularly among Emergency Medicine physicians. This part of the application was painful to complete, but I gave the full details as requested.

After the usual vetting process I was accepted to the Bozeman Hospital staff. As to my gig on *Consenting Adults Only*, it never came up. I figured most Montanans are not in Gabe Stein's demographic.

We planned to move the first week of September.

CHAPTER 36

IN EARLY AUGUST I RECEIVED my expert's deposition in the mail, with a cover letter from Attorney Randall asking me please read it, then give him a call.

Dr. Steve Davis is an ED physician in Reno's leading medical center. I don't know him, have never met him, which is a good thing since you don't want a friend to defend you; it looks too cozy to the jury. The plaintiff's attorney would point it out in a millisecond.

Dr. Davis's deposition began like mine, with the usual questions from Mr. Gramble about medical training and current position, and if he had reviewed the records in this case.

A: Yes, I have.
Q: Have you discussed this case with Dr. Luvkin?
A: No, I have not.
Q: Have you discussed this case with any other physicians?
A: No, I have not.
Q: Is it the standard of care to rule out an acute heart problem in a patient who presents to the ED with chest pain?
A: Yes.
Q: Is it the standard of care to do an EKG in this type of patient?
A: Yes.
Q: Is it the standard of care to order cardiac enzymes?
A: Yes.

Q: Can these tests be negative and the patient still have major
coronary artery disease?
A: Yes

Of course, I read all this with more interest than a John Grisham novel,
since every answer could impact my fate. So far it seemed to be boiler-
plate medical questions, but I sensed a trap was being set. I was right.

Q: If that possibility exists, then is it appropriate to proceed with
a stress test?

Wow! I could see the trap. Attorney Gramble changed from "standard
of care" to "appropriate." If he got Dr. Davis to answer a simple "yes"
then he would quote him back to the jury. "But you said it was appropriate to do a stress test. Was one done?"

Never mind that no time frame was mentioned, or anything about
clinical judgment. Attorney Gramble would have Dr. Davis on record
admitting it's appropriate to do the stress test. If in trial Dr. Davis tried
to qualify an answer, Gramble could first insist on a yes or no, then let
him explain, but the damage would be done. The jury would hear "yes"
and might not be interested in any further explanation.

The smart expert isn't caught by this attorney trick. Davis was smart.

A: I'm sorry, I don't understand your question. What do you mean
by possibility?
Q: "Well, if the patient could have significant heart disease, and it
could be determined by a stress test, would it be appropriate to do
the test sooner rather than later."
A: I'm sorry. I'm not trying to be difficult, here. But it's possible
anyone at any time could have heart disease. It's neither practical
nor advisable to do an immediate stress test on every patient who
presents to the ED with chest pain. It's certainly not the standard
of care. You have to use some clinical judgment about if and when
a stress test is done.

So Dr. Davis did not fall for the trap and Gramble changed course. After an hour of back and forth haggling, Gramble said, "I have no further questions."

My attorney had a few, to get Dr. Davis's formal opinion on the record.

Mr. Randall: Based on your background, training and knowledge, do you have an opinion as to whether Dr. Luvkin met the standard of care in treating Mr. Steiger the date of his ED visit?
Q: I do.
Mr. Randall: And what is that opinion?
A: My opinion is that he met the standard of care.
Mr. Randall: Thank you. No further questions.

As with the other two depositions, the hospital's attorney had to get his two cents in. After the usual introduction Attorney Bigsby asked:

Q. Doctor, do you find any fault with the hospital in this case. By hospital, I mean its employees, or policies?
A. No, none at all.
Q. Thank you. No further questions.

I called Attorney Randall after reading the deposition. He was upbeat.

"Dr. Davis is a savvy expert, Josh. It was a good deposition."

"It certainly seems so."

"Gramble still fully intends to go to trial. He's got his expert witness and a dead patient, and of course the wife's testimony."

"Which is?"

"Did I send you her deposition?"

"I don't think so."

"I think I mentioned this before. Basically, she's claiming that her multiple sclerosis worsened after he died, and there's no way she can go out and work. That's going to generate some jury sympathy. Doesn't even need a doctor to verify, it's all subjective."

"Did he have life insurance?"

"Yes, but that's not admissible in court. Policy was only seventy-five thousand."

"And the claim is for one million?"

"Right."

"And her attorney will get forty percent of that?"

"Josh, I don't think you should worry about the attorney here. Mr. Gramble is not the plaintiff, and the jury is never going to not give an award because the attorney will get rich off it. Jurors don't think that way."

"No, I understand. Actually, I feel sorry for her. I just don't think I fell below any standard of care, and don't want this on my record when I don't think I did anything wrong.

Can a jury decide malpractice based on the widow's circumstances? I mean, shouldn't it be based on the medical alone?"

"Yes, and I'm going to argue that none of her social and economic status be admissible, such as her monthly expenses. But the judge will allow Gramble to ask about the impact of her husband's sudden demise, and she's going to say her MS got worse as a result, that she wishes she could work but can't. The judge isn't going to strike that. So it's subtle, but Gramble's going to get as much in as he can. Legally, though, if the jury doesn't feel there is any malpractice, she won't get a dime. The problem is, if they do, her story can affect the award."

"This is making my head spin," I said. "I say we go to trial." I was firm, and saw no reason to settle this case.

"Then we agree. So in trial, all I want you to do is focus on the medical, and try not to let your anger about the legal system manifest. Also, don't say you feel sorry for her. Just stay medical and let me worry about the tactics, and how we're going to argue this. Of course, just before the trial we'll meet and I'll go over this in much more detail."

"That's fine. Thanks for the advice, but I think you can see how a case like this can affect someone."

"I see it in every case, and always give the same advice. Stay calm, stick to the medical,

and don't wear any anger or emotions on your sleeve."

———

Just two weeks before we were to leave Vegas, my ED colleague Bill Munson returned from a trip to San Francisco, where he attended the Western States Convention of Emergency Medicine physicians. I didn't go for two reasons. One, it was close to our moving time. You can guess the other.

"Met a colleague of yours at the convention," he said.

"Oh?"

"Yeah, a gal named Judy Berkowitz, says she knows you from medical school and you briefly dated."

"Briefly? Anything else?"

"Still seems interested in you. Asked a lot of questions."

"Yeah, we dated briefly. Nothing came of it. Did you tell her I'm moving?"

"Well, yeah, I didn't think it was a secret. But she did ask."

"What exactly did you tell her?"

"Just that you were moving up north. I'm not even sure where. Is it Utah, Wyoming? I remember someplace up north. Hope I didn't spill any beans."

I tried hard to not show my angst over this latest development. "Nah," I said. "She's one of those busybody reunion gals, always wants to stay on top of where our classmates are. I'm sure I'll hear from her at some point. Frankly, she's kind of obnoxious, always wants to know what you're doing with your life. She was the same in medical school. Kind of a chatterbox."

"So where *are* you going?" Bill asked.

"Montana. But if by any chance she calls to find out, tell her Maine, OK?"

"Yeah, sure."

———

We counted down the days. The heat in August was stifling and made us long for the drive to Montana.

It had been a rough year. I had survived Judy's craziness, the local newspapers, the hospital's bylaws, and had not given in to the meritless lawsuit. I was on the good side of Gabe and Jack, and probably also Carl, though as expected we had no further contact with him after Irene left town.

My parents now fully accepted Barbara into the family and looked forward to their third grandchild. About Montana, not so much.

"It's cold in Montana," Mom said over the phone.

"Mom, it's cold where you live, in case you haven't noticed."

"But Montana's far away."

"We'll visit."

"Promise?"

"Promise."

"You know, when you went to Yellowstone before your senior year in college, I was worried you'd be attacked by a bear. Did you know that?"

"No, you never told me. I only saw two bears the whole summer. And they were at a distance."

"It's my anxiety, Josh, I know, but stay away from bears in Montana."

"I will Mom, I promise."

The only thorn in our leaving was the upcoming trial; I still had to return for it. With travel time, this meant at least a week away from home, the same week as Barbara's due date. She was accepting, but not happy with the coincidence.

"You have to do what you have to do. It's a onetime thing. We'll survive. I'll have Mom come that week."

"And what if we have the child the week before?"

"Josh, she's retired. She'll come when she has to."

"It'll be cold."

"Seattle is not exactly Miami Beach in January."

"This is a real bummer, the more I think about it. We don't know anyone in Montana, you're due mid-January, and I'm due then also. For a different venue."

"Are you changing your mind?"

"Perhaps. I need to think on it."

———————

One day in late-August I drove to Red Rock Canyon and hiked Oak Creek trail. It is less traveled than the other Red Rock trails, and gives sweeping views of the Red Rock escarpment. It was hot but I didn't mind. I took a wide sombrero type hat to protect against the sun and plenty of water. The main thing, is, I had space and time to think. I sat on a rock and weighed all the pros and cons of going to trial or settling.

There was no way I could be out of town when our baby was born. There was also no way I wanted to settle this case, which would forever be on my record for any medical application of any sort. I felt as if Attorney Gramble had a chain around my neck and could yank it at any time. Without Gramble and this awful lawsuit, I was a free man. With him and his lust for a fat payday, I was a prisoner. Mrs. Steiger was the plaintiff but my wrath was for her attorney and the legal system.

I drove home and called Attorney Randall. He knew we were leaving town, of course, but not the actual date.

"We're moving next week. Is the trial still in January?"

"Yes, it is. You'll have to come back."

"My baby is due the same week. Can it be postponed a month?"

"Possibly. That is an extenuating circumstance. I assume you'd have no trouble getting a medical letter to confirm the date?"

"No, of course not."

"Well, if you want me to try, I'll do so. Gramble can object of course, but in the end it's up to the judge. I think we have a shot at one postponement, but that would be it. If there's a problem with your wife's health, or the baby's, I don't think we could get a second delay. Just letting you know."

Now I had visions of the baby being born with a heart defect, or Barbara having post-partum depression and needing me close to her. I knew too much medical stuff and envisioned all the worst. Why do I want to take this risk? My mind turned over all the possibilities.

"Doctor, are you there?"

"Yes, yes, I'm just thinking."

"Let me call you back tomorrow," I said. "This is a difficult decision to make."

"No problem. Call me tomorrow"

I knew what Barbara would want. So much so, it was not even fair to discuss the issue any further with her. That night I wrestled in bed with my options. Go to Vegas in January? Postpone the trial, perhaps to February or March? Continue with this noose around my neck?

I kissed my wife and tried to sleep. Sleep was fitful and I dragged the next day at work. I did not call Mr. Randall then. Or the following day.

Barbara was beginning to show quite a bit. Ultrasounds revealed the baby was fine. She went looking for a crib and other baby items, but decided not to buy anything until we settled in Bozeman.

Meanwhile, I bought the gun. I went to Gold and Silver Pawn, because it was convenient and also because I was curious to see the locale of History Channel's hit show *Pawn Stars*. The "Stars" were not there of course but seeing the store with its mob of customers was still a treat. After a couple of inquiries, and making it clear this was my first purchase and I knew zilch about guns, I was connected with a knowledgeable salesman. He suggested the not-inexpensive Glock 43, a 9-mm pistol. It felt good in my hand.

After the required background check I bought the gun and went to a shooting range twice over the next several days. It was not difficult to use and, I must admit, felt empowering. I hoped I would never need it.

With some trepidation, I asked Barbara if she wanted to learn. Her reaction was instant.

"You bought a gun? Are you serious? No way. I might use it." She really had no interest and I didn't push it.

———◆———

It was near the end of August and we were to leave in a week for Montana. I wanted to decide the malpractice issue before then. Four days after my last discussion with Attorney Randall I called again.

"I've decided."

"Let's have it."

"I never want to return here."

"What are you saying?"

"See if you can settle. I'm not going for any postponement. I might win at trial, I might lose. It's a gamble, like everything else in this god-forsaken town. I am not a gambler. At least no more. I need to get on with my life. Can you do this with Bigsby, make a package offer? Maybe half a million? Gramble will clear a couple hundred thousand, for what I imagine was not a whole lot of work. He should be satisfied."

"Are you sure?"

"About as sure as anything else. The thought of coming back to the Clark County Courthouse keeps me up at night. Not to mention my lovely wife. There's just too much going on. I am not going to leave her in the middle of a Montana winter, when we are expecting."

"I understand. It's your call, Josh. If settling is what you want, I'll arrange a meeting with Gramble and Bigsby. I'll tell them you're leaving the state. However, in point of fact you really don't have to be present in a civil case. I can represent you without your physical presence."

"But you wouldn't want to, I'm sure."

"Not a good idea. The jury sees an empty chair, they might figure you've got something to hide. I could introduce your wife's maternity, but Gramble then could make a stink, arguing that you could have asked for a postponement. Worse, he could paint a picture to the jury of you as arrogant, uncaring and flippant."

"Yeah, he would do that, I'm sure."

"Without you there to show them what a nice guy you really are, it would be difficult to counter a negative image. I know you want this case adjudicated on the medical facts, but I've got to tell you, a negative image can sway jurors on the fence. So it's never a good way to handle a trial. But as your attorney it's an option I have to make you aware of."

"I appreciate what you're telling me. Clearly not showing up seems like a sure way to lose big. Talk to Gramble and Bigsby. See what happens."

"OK, I'll get back to you. By the way, why Montana? You like snow?"

"Not especially. But the air is clean, and the people are too. No offense, just that my wife and I need a change of scenery."

"I'll get back to you."

———◆———

Mr. Randall called back a few days later.

"Good news, sort of."

"I'm listening."

"The widow will settle for $650,000. I think they know they have a weak case medically, and she's afraid of losing. Your insurance company will pay $500,000 and the hospital will put up $150,000.

My heart sank. Not such good news. The higher the number, the more culpability I was made to feel.

"What do you think?" I asked.

"Doctor…" He sometimes called me doctor to emphasize the professional relationship. "…I'm prepared to go to trial. At this point it's up to you. I don't think she'll go any lower."

"I really have no choice," I said. "Let's settle the case."

Almost immediately I felt relieved and saddened. Life is full of ups and downs and this was a downer, but I would get over it. Looking back, I don't think I made the wrong decision.

———◆———

Jack Strawn and I had a few conversations over the summer. His arraignment for the state was scheduled for August 25th. The federal case would be adjudicated after Nevada was through with him. He was at risk for up to five years in jail, because of all the documented activity at Joes Plumbing and the one prior felony conviction for wife battery. He didn't know what extra jail time there might be from not paying taxes, since that was a federal charge. At this point he only had a state public defender and was not optimistic.

As to the other contest participants, he said "they got stuff against all of us." He thought Joe the plumber had his own private attorney. "Joe will be long dead before they put him away" was his insightful comment.

The arraignment day came and went and Jack did not appear. I did not know this at the time, and merely waited on Jack's promised phone call to keep me informed. After two days without a call I contacted the public defender, told him I had posted Jack's bond and asked what happened.

"Are you a relative?"

"No, no, just good friend."

"I'm very sorry, sir," he said.

"About what? What happened?"

"Mr. Strawn is dead. Apparent suicide. They found his body at the bottom of Angel Cliff the day after his arraignment. He was in his car, crushed by the impact. Ran it off the road. I'm afraid his case is closed."

"Thank you, I didn't know. I didn't know. Was there a note?"

"Actually, there was. It was short. It said, 'I'm tired of this shit'. That's all."

I thanked him, hung up the phone and cried.

———◆———

We left town on Labor Day, with Barbara four and a half months pregnant. The first few miles were the most difficult. We drove right past the Lindholm Hotel, still closed for reconstruction. It was scheduled to re-open by the end of the year. The perpetrators had been identified as of Middle Eastern origin but were yet unnamed. Two Islamic groups claimed responsibility. Investigation focused on possible accomplices. The final death toll was now 102.

"Do you think people will stay there when it reopens?" Barbara asked.

"I suppose so. If the price is right. It could happen anywhere, any time."

"Bozeman?"

"No, not Bozeman. Probably the least likely place to be hit by terrorists. Bozeman is at risk for another catastrophe, far, far worse."

"I know, you've told me. The Yellowstone Caldera."

"Yep. When Yellowstone blows, it really won't matter much where you live within a thousand miles."

"And remind me one more time when this is supposed to occur?"

"Half a million years, give or take a hundred thousand."

Thoughts of Armageddon were interrupted on Interstate 15 when we hit a major traffic snarl, still inside the city limits. A truck had jack-knifed and traffic slowed to a crawl for a good half hour while police tried to clear a lane.

"I guess they don't want us to leave Vegas," Barbara said.

"Looks that way."

Once moving again we passed the Leaving Las Vegas sign, almost an hour after starting out. It was then I remembered what Carl had said the night of our wedding, regarding Judy's appearance at the hotel and the subsequent showdown with Gil Perkins: *he doesn't think you and Barbara will be bothered any longer. At least not in Las Vegas.* And we had not been, at least not with any personal appearances. And since Judy's Michelangelo statue, not one package or letter had arrived from her hand, not one text message. She had met my colleague Bill Munson in San Francisco, and then only made what to him seemed like innocent inquiry.

Had she found another boyfriend? Had the LVPD and LAPD threats worked? Was she done with me? Or was she sitting back, plotting and planning? I even wondered if perhaps she had placed a GPS device on my car, and had the car checked before we left; none was found. All these thoughts went through my head as we headed north. If she was still in California, and I was no longer in Vegas, what could she do? And for what gain? Why would she want to? It made no sense. And that was the rub. It made no sense *to me.*

We hit the open road, no houses, no development, just nature of the American Southwest.

"It feels good to get on the highway," Barbara said. "Isn't the desert beautiful?"

"Yes, in its own way. But I'm looking forward to deep forests, wide rivers and greenery."

"Well, let's hurry, before it all turns white."

We drove north, braced for the coming winter and a new life in Big Sky Country.

CHAPTER 37

———◆———

ONE OF MY FAVORITE HIKES in Yellowstone Park is Point Sublime. During my summer job I had hiked it twice, starting from Artist's point. The path is well traveled in the warm months, but much less so in the fall, by which time most of the park's tourists have vanished.

One weekend in late October the sky was clear blue, the prediction for a crisp forty-five degrees in the afternoon. I was off for the day. Barbara's mother was visiting from Seattle, helping her prepare for our new child. I decided to drive to Artist's Point and hike Point Sublime.

The drive took ninety minutes. There were only a couple of cars in the parking lot, and some picture-takers viewing the Lower Falls. The hike to Point Sublime leads away from the Lower Falls and borders the steep valley gorged by the Yellowstone River. It is a about a mile one way and I figured to do the two-mile round trip in an hour, including a stop at the Point to take in the view. I wanted to reminisce about my summer at Old Faithful Lodge.

As you walk the path, on your left the river is 1000 feet down a steeply sloping canyon wall. On your right, the woods are thick and in some places take a steep ascent. The man-made path is reasonably wide, well laid out, and there is little danger of falling if you stick to it. I carried a small backpack, with some water, nut mix, bear spray, jacket, and a regular camera in case my smart phone camera acted up. Also in the backpack was my Glock 43, loaded, with the safety lock on.

I saw no one on the hike out. The wind rustled, the river far below flowed silently, and I was thinking nature. Another month or so and the path would close due to snow and ice, but now it was picture- and sound-perfect. I reached the Point, a small clearing surrounded by a wooden railing overlooking the river. I leaned over the railing and took some pictures. I thought back to my Midwest upbringing, the years of medical training, my short career at Memorial Hospital, and life now with Barbara and the coming of fatherhood. Montana and Wyoming fit just right. I was glad to be free of all the craziness in Las Vegas.

I started back. In less than a minute I saw a figure walking toward me. Another hiker on this lonely, scenic trail. The hiker at first looked vaguely familiar. She was smiling, waving. "Hello," she called out, as if she knew me. As we drew closer I strained to make her out. It was Judy, and I instantly knew. This was no coincidence.

I am an emergency medicine doctor, trained to spot crises and react quickly. I am also a nice guy, with a family and a career and a full life ahead. My stalker had caught up with me, in the serenity and loneliness of this path. I had one thought: *I don't deserve this. I know what she wants.*

"Judy? Is that you?"

She stopped about thirty yards away. She held something in her right hand. A gun.

On my right was the canyon. On my left, a steep rocky wall. No place to run or hide.

"I can't believe I met you here, Josh. What a coincidence."

If I stood and talked, I would be an easy target. If I turned and ran, my back would be to her, also an easy target. And if I went for the Glock, then what?

The gun's in the bottom of my backpack. What if I fumble inside and can't get it out in time? What if she sees the gun and starts shooting before I can even aim the thing? And could I even aim it accurately and pull the trigger? And if I could, do I have it in me to kill another person? What if she has a toy pistol and she's just playing a prank, and I kill her? Or if I shoot and miss, and her gun is real?

"Judy, I have something for you," I said, and began removing my backpack. "I've been meaning to give it to you."

"You do?" she said. My offer caught her by surprise, enough to distract her momentarily.

I swung the back pack around and held it tightly to my chest, then began running toward her, keeping to my left, as far from the canyon drop off as possible.

She was caught off guard by my sudden rushing forward. She raised her right hand and fired.

Bam! Bam!

Both shots missed. By the time I reached her she was yelling, "You son of a bitch! You son of a bitch!" I threw the back pack hard at her and she tripped back, near the path's edge. I jumped on top and tried wrestling the gun from her right hand, but she held it tightly. She was stronger than I expected. She spit in my eyes and I momentarily lost my grip. She scooted from underneath me and tried to regain her balance, gun still in hand. She seemed unaware of her position on the path and stood perilously close to the rim, about four feet from my head. I saw her raise the gun barrel. I had to act fast. I leaped at her feet before she could fire, grabbed her ankles hard and she fell backwards, so that her torso and hips hung below the edge of the canyon wall. Only her lower legs rested on the path, kept there by the strength of my double grip. I dug my hiking shoes into the dirt path to keep from sliding and held her ankles tightly.

"Josh, I'm falling!" she yelled. "I'm falling! Help me!"

I turned my head to look around, did not see her gun.

"Pull me up, Josh! Pull me up! I'll be a good girl, I promise. Pull me up! Pleeeze!"

It might be possible. Holding on to her ankles, the toes of my shoes dug into the dirt path. If I crawled over her legs and reached over with one arm, I might be able to pull her up, but would have little leverage and the action might also drag me over the edge. We both could be killed. And if I was successful, then what? More of the same? Barbara next time? I had to make a decision.

I let go. She took the gun with her.

Epilogue

I CALLED A PARK RANGER as soon as I reached cell phone service, which was near sunset. I explained the encounter, how Judy fell backward over the cliff and when I looked down I could not see her body. The first 200 feet are sheer vertical cliff, and beyond that a sharp slope into a grove of trees. There was no way she could have survived. My story quickly escalated up the chain of command. The rangers all agreed it was too late to start searching for her body. Just before sunset they closed off Point Sublime to all hikers.

The next morning a helicopter surveyed the area below the lookout and spotted her body among some trees. There is no place to land in that part of the canyon so retrieval had to come from above, by rappelling down the cliff. A team of rangers experienced in mountain rescues was called in. They found her horribly mangled body some 250 feet below the path. The gun was nowhere near and the rangers didn't spend a lot of time looking for it. Their immediate challenge was to bring back the body, for autopsy and then burial.

Did I commit a crime? Of course not. She tried to kill me and I defended myself. But without the gun I was a suspect. There were no grounds yet for any charge, but the nature of the rangers' questions made it clear I was not off the hook. They expressed surprise that a young woman physician would go to all the trouble of traveling from California to Wyoming, and with a gun no less. Perhaps they would have preferred a more plausible story, like maybe I lured Judy to Point Sublime and then pushed her off the path to get rid of her. This scenario wasn't offered -- they are park rangers, not police investigators -- but still I felt their skepticism.

I did not mess around and hired a Bozeman criminal attorney, Craig Stark. My third attorney in a year: malpractice, contract, criminal. I was keeping the law profession busy.

The FBI took charge of the investigation since the park is federal land. They interviewed me twice, both times with Mr. Stark at my side. I provided every detail, save one: that I *might* have been able to pull Judy back up. All I said was that I grabbed her ankles but could not hold on.

My attorney secured Judy's files from LVPD and LAPD, and with that information convinced the FBI agents that Judy was intent on harm and that the gun was a crucial piece of evidence. Of course the FBI did its own investigation, first of Judy's car at Artist's Point parking lot, then of her cell phone. In the phone they found GPS software used to track another vehicle. Mine. Then they searched my car and found a magnetized signaler underneath, probably put there when I was working in the Bozeman ED.

The agents also learned Judy had spent the previous two nights in a Bozeman motel, registered under the name under Judy Schuster. She had a piece of ID with that name from when she was married. My stalker may have been unbalanced, but she was also smart and resourceful.

With all this information, the FBI directed the Yellowstone rangers to go back and find the gun. This was a problem since it could be almost anywhere above or below where she landed. Fortunately the location precluded the gun ever being moved or picked up by any hikers.

Two rangers rappelled down to look for the gun. Luckily, after an hour of searching they found it, about fifty yards from where she landed. Forensic analysis discovered Judy's fingerprints and none of mine, and confirmed the firing of two bullets. Everything fit with the details of my story. There was a hearing a week later before a federal judge in Cheyenne. After an hour I was fully exonerated of any crime. Judy's death was ruled "accidental."

I was not done yet. Bozeman is a small city and the publicity was unnerving. "Woman falls to death in Yellowstone after spat with local doctor," read one headline. "FBI investigating Yellowstone death. Local doctor cooperating," and "Doctor Luvkin judged innocent in Yellowstone hiker's death" read two others. I was repeatedly called for interviews, comments. On the advice of my attorney I spoke to no one about the case. Even my parents, who called every night that first week, had to make do with "Everything's fine, don't worry, can't go into any details." I gave a similar response to my colleagues at work. I confided to just two people during this ordeal, Barbara and Craig Stark.

Since I was innocent, a victim of sorts myself, there was no basis for any hospital action. No calls to the CEO's office, no PQC meeting. Actually, most of the hospital staff were sympathetic, not just because I had been stalked by a crazy woman, but also because Barbara worked there and was pregnant. After a few weeks things were almost back to normal.

But not quite. One more hurdle. Judy's mother sued me in civil court for "causing the death of her daughter." Civil suits have a much lower threshold for evidence than a criminal case. I had already been around the block with a meritless malpractice lawsuit, and was not going to lie down for this one. Mr. Stark agreed to defend it, since he already knew all the details.

The suit was filed in Montana State Court in Helena; this was permissible since I lived in the state and Yellowstone Park spills over into Montana. I had never met her mother, and didn't want to. She hired a local attorney who no doubt envisioned easy settlement dollars in his bank account. I was prepared to go bankrupt to defend this suit.

We countersued, both Judy's mother *and* her attorney for frivolous litigation. We cited the LVPD and LAPD reports. We submitted affidavits obtained from Gil Perkins, Carl Collins and Sergeant Nelson. I was pleased that Carl had no objection when Attorney Stark called him. Stark told me the Las Vegas trio already knew about Judy's death and in general "were not surprised." So we had all this documentation, plus the FBI investigation report. Stark also threatened publicity about Judy's mental instability (her letter to me, the Michelangelo statue "gift"), and how all this might impact the plaintiff (her mother) when the news got out. Then he filed a detailed motion for dismissal.

It was a battle of attorneys. Mrs. Berkowitz's Helena lawyer was in a bind. He had accepted the case not knowing all the details, and now was himself a defendant. I went to the hearing for dismissal, held before State Judge Gretchen Demora. The judge asked plaintiff's attorney on what grounds Mrs. Berkowitz sought civil damages. His answers were vague, assumptive: "wrongful death"; "she didn't have to die"; "there is no evidence she fired those bullets at Dr. Luvkin."

"Was she squirrel hunting, then?" asked the judge. I loved it. Plaintiff's attorney had no answer.

My attorney was a tad more eloquent, stating "my client suffered significantly at the hands of the deceased. While all deaths are tragic, and loss of a child particularly so, it would be grossly unfair to proceed with a civil action in the face of overwhelming evidence that no crime was committed, and that Dr. Luvkin acted in self-defense. We sincerely believe this suit is without merit and intend to defend it vigorously, your honor. For the record, I have filed separate motions against both the plaintiff and her lawyer, for instigating a lawsuit they know to be without merit."

Judge Demora ordered everyone to return the next day. In the meantime she would review all the documents. I had to work at the hospital, so couldn't attend.

The following day Attorney Stark called. "Case dismissed," he said. "The judge agreed the civil case was without merit, and she wasn't going to waste taxpayer money letting it proceed to jury trial." At that, my lawyer withdrew our countersuits. He also told me that plaintiff's attorney seemed visibly relieved at the judge's decision.

My total legal bill since Judy's attack: $27,000. I did not begrudge the expense. My attorney was worth every penny.

Barbara weathered all this beautifully. In a little over a year we had been through so much together. "You know," I said, "we should write a book about all that's happened to us. When I first called Dr. Siegel in Vegas to set up an appointment, she even thought our story sounded like a novel. And that was before Judy attacked me."

"Write a book?" she asked. *"Another* side job?"

"Just a thought," I said.

"Let's keep it that way," she replied.

On the last day of January, Barbara gave birth to Melissa Deborah Luvkin, eight pounds, five ounces. Normal delivery, healthy baby. Everything went well. The next day I brought Barbara and Melissa home.

For the first time in over a year I had no entanglements, no lawyers and no outside pressures. Best of all, I now had my own family. Life was good.

THE END

www.ingramcontent.com/pod-product-compliance
Lightning Source LLC
Chambersburg PA
CBHW060006210326
41520CB00009B/834